Early communicative skills

Early communicative skills

Gilbert MacKay
and
William Dunn

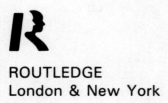

ROUTLEDGE
London & New York

First published 1989
by Routledge
11 New Fetter Lane, London EC4P 4EE
29 West 35th Street, New York, NY 10001

Phototypeset in 10pt Times by
Mews Photosetting, Beckenham, Kent
Printed and bound in Great Britain by Mackays of Chatham PLC, Kent

British Library Cataloguing in Publication Data

MacKay, Gilbert, *1944–*
    Early communicative skills.
    1. Mentally handicapped children.
    Communication. Teaching.
    I. Title II. Dunn, William.
    371.92′8
    ISBN 0-415-03204-0
    ISBN 0-415-03205-9 (pbk.)

Library of Congress Cataloging-in-Publication Data

MacKay, Gilbert, 1944–
    Early communicative skills / Gilbert MacKay and William Dunn.
        p.   cm.
    Bibliography: p.
    Includes index.
    ISBN 0-415-03204-0 ISBN 0-415-03205-9 (pbk.)
    1. Learning disabled children–Language. 2. Learning disabled
children–Education–Language arts. 3. Oral Communication–Study
and teaching. 4. Communicative disorders in children. I. Dunn,
William. II. Title.
    LC4704.85.M33   1989
    371.9′044–dc19   88-30772
                                                            CIP

To Isobel, Seonaid, and Finlay

Contents

Illustrations   x

Tables   xi

Acknowledgement   xii

Introduction   1

Part 1   The development of communication   13

Stage 1: The children have profound learning difficulties   15

Stage 2: The children begin to take an active interest in
their surroundings   17

Stage 3: The children begin to understand words and gestures   19

Stage 4: The children produce their own first words   21

Stage 5: The children use connected speech   23

Part 2   Activities for developing communication   25

Stimulating hearing   27

Stimulating vision   41

Stimulating the sense of touch   49

Stimulating the sense of movement   57

Stimulating the sense of smell   67

Stimulating the sense of taste   75

Watching and finding things   77

Handling objects   87

Contents

Behaving purposefully 109

Making things happen 121

Understanding the positioning of objects 131

Recognizing and understanding sounds 141

Imitating actions 155

Imitating vocal sounds 164

Make-believe play 168

Understanding words 176

Producing first words 191

More advanced understanding of language 212

Producing more advanced language 225

Language without speech 238

Beyond two-word sentences 243

Part 3 Problems in the development of communication 245

Children who do not appear to be conscious 247

Children who do not handle or play with objects 248

Children who lose interest in objects after they have been removed
from view 249

Children who show few signs of purposeful behaviour 251

Children who do not understand that there are reasons that
events occur 253

Children who do not understand the importance of the positioning of
objects 255

Children who are unable to imitate the sounds or the actions of other
people 257

Children who do not take part in make-believe, imaginative play 259

Children who do not understand language 261

Children who do not produce single words 263

Children who use single words but not connected speech 265

Withdrawn children   267

Children who have difficulty in forming relationships with people   269

Children who are overactive   271

Children who are easily distracted   272

Children who behave impulsively   273

Children who keep repeating a word or action after it has served its
     purpose for them   274

Echolalia, or 'echoed speech'   275

Cocktail-party speech   277

Part 4 Record-keeping   279

Day-sheet   281

Word-record   283

Frequency-record   286

References   289

Index   292

Illustrations

1 Rocking-board   60

2 Down Box   199

3 Goodbye-Hello Box   199

4 Paget-Gorman sign for 'orange'   239

5 Day-sheet   282

6 Word-record   284

7 Word-record   285

8 Frequency-record   288

Tables

1 Functions of single-word utterances   4
2 The five stages of Early Communicative Skills   5
3 The six sensorimotor actions identified by Piaget   7
4 General teaching aims for the five stages   8
5 Relating the five stages to teaching activities   9
6 Target words for noun/pronoun comprehension   177
7 A basis for increased understanding   212
8 A basis for vocabulary-building   215
9 Early descriptive vocabulary   221

Acknowledgement

This manual is based on a mimeograph produced by the authors at the Department of Education, University of Glasgow. The mimeograph was the major outcome of the Early Communicative Skills Project which was located at the Department of Education, University of Glasgow, and funded by the Scottish Education Department and the Mental Health Foundation.

Introduction

A framework for communication   3

Using *Early communicative skills*   10

What? No assessment charts?   11

Introduction

A framework for communication

Communication is a basic human need. It lets people form and maintain relationships through the sharing of thoughts, feelings, wants, and intentions. People who have difficulty in communicating may therefore be excluded, accidentally or deliberately, from the social exchanges of everyday life. This is why communication has an important place in the curriculum of all school pupils, irrespective of their age and ability. Nowhere is its place more important than in the curriculum of pupils who have difficulty in learning. This manual has been written with one such group of pupils in mind, those with severe and profound learning difficulties.

Children with severe and profound learning difficulties acquired the same right to education as every other child by Education Acts in England and Wales (1970) and Scotland (1974). Their difficulties with learning present the educational system with many challenges. Providing these pupils with experiences in the area of communication is one of the most important challenges, because delayed or disordered communication is a principal characteristic of severe and profound learning difficulty.

The manual aims to respond to the need to communicate of pupils who have not yet reached the level of speaking in two-word sentences. This level is normally reached by children when they are about two-and-a-half years old. The first two-and-a-half years are a short period in the span of human development, but the range of communicative competence within them is considerable among pupils with learning difficulties as a result of the wide spread of ages, experience, physical difficulties, personalities, and other individual characteristics.

Restricting the area of communication to be covered to such an early part of the developmental range also has implications for how we think about communication. Normally there is little wrong with describing communication as *what happens when people talk and listen to each other*. However, that description is not very useful when people have no speech or any other system of language such as writing or hand-signs. And, of course, communication may occur in the absence of language. For example, parents recognize that they and their infant

3

children are able to communicate long before the children are able to talk. Indeed, studies of mother–child interaction have shown that complex exchanges, the roots of communication, have begun to occur in the early weeks, and even days, after birth (Trevarthen 1977).

Teasing out the essence of communication is beyond the scope of this manual, though it is dealt with in many texts on psycholinguistics, communication theory, and philosophy. Here a simple, perhaps simplistic, description of communication as *the sharing of ideas* or *the exchange of messages* will suffice. The advantage of this description is that, though it certainly encompasses communication by speech, hand-signs, writing, and any other language, language is not implicit in it. There is a place in it for gesture, crying, tugging, or any activity which makes one person behave as if the person in action is trying to convey a message. It therefore can accommodate the entire range of pupils whose level of communication is at or below the two-word stage.

How, then, may pupils learn to share ideas or exchange messages? One useful approach is to look at the routines of effective communication which grow out of the interaction of mothers and children. *Let's Talk* (McConkey and Price 1986) is an example of this approach, containing excellent ideas on how parents and teachers may encourage the development of children's communication by responding to their spontaneous and elicited activity.

Early communicative skills takes a different, but complementary, view of communication. It is not concerned with answering the question 'How do people communicate?', but rather with 'Why do they communicate?', or 'What purposes does communication serve for them?' This question has interested British psycholinguists for more than a decade. For instance, M.A.K. Halliday (1975) noted that the first words of his son could be classified as the functions which appear in table 1.

Table 1 Functions of single-word utterances (based on Halliday 1975)

Function	Purpose	Example in adult language
Instrumental	Satisfies speaker's needs	'I want . . . '
Regulatory	Controls others	'Do this'
Interactional	Fosters relationships	'Hello'
Personal	Expresses own uniqueness	'Here is what I think'
Heuristic	Increases knowledge	'Tell me why . . . '
Imaginative	Creates own world of make-believe	'Let's pretend . . . '
Informative	Recounts experiences	'I've something to tell you'

And Joan Tough, using a similar set of purposes, has based techniques for fostering the communicative development of young children (Tough 1976, 1977) and of pupils with moderate learning difficulties (Tough 1981) on the premise that the purposefulness of communication is a key to how it may be taught.

Now, it is easy to talk about the purposes of communication for people who can talk, but is it so reasonable to look for purpose in the communicative acts of children before they have acquired speech? Parents of young children would say that it is, for they become adept at interpreting messages of hunger, pleasure, discomfort, and so on in their children's actions and vocalizations before the onset of speech. Indeed it has been shown that a wide range of communicative purposes, such as those described by Halliday and Tough, may be observed in the actions of infants who have yet to begin to speak (Dore 1975). We would like to suggest that the sequence of communicative development between birth and two-word sentences may be divided into a series of stages which give direction to the teaching of communication. The scheme has its origins in a description of the development of vocal sounds (Nakazima 1975), but it has been modified and expanded to make it more appropriate as a guide to activities for teaching and learning.

Five stages are described to chart the development of communication up to the two-word level. These stages are summarized in table 2.

Table 2 The five stages of early communicative skills

Stage	Description
1	Children with the most profound learning difficulties. They rarely or never act spontaneously and may often seem to be asleep.
2	Children who have begun to take an active interest in their surroundings, but who do not understand or use speech.
3	Children who understand some words; children who have begun to imitate words.
4	Children who speak single words.
5	Children who use connected speech.

Stage 1 is concerned with children at the earliest developmental levels and therefore with those who have the most profound learning difficulties. Their level of functioning is early in what the Swiss psychologist, Jean Piaget, called the 'sensorimotor' stage of development. By this he meant that the dominant influences on the intellectual development of children at this stage (in the first and second years of life) are sensory stimulation ('sensori') and action ('motor').

Children at Stage 1 in our scheme are functioning mainly at the sensory level because the severity of their difficulties restricts their capacity for movement and other activity. What is the purpose of communication for them? If they are not active, they will be unable to produce deliberate actions and vocalizations which other people may interpret as messages. However, the 'sensori' of 'sensorimotor' is also important. If we want them to communicate, or 'share ideas', as best they can, then they must have ideas to share, and these ideas are provided by sensory stimulation in the first place. This is why stimulation of the senses has an established place in schemes of activities for children with the most profound degrees of difficulty, those who often seem to spend a large part of their lives asleep. Credit for much pioneering work in the area of sensory stimulation in Britain is due to Mildred Stevens (1976), and some of the ideas which appear in Part 3 of the manual have their origins in her work with children in the north-west of England.

It is also important to remember, when working with children at Stage 1, that communication has two types of participants: those who transmit messages and those who receive them. The child may appear to have no messages to transmit to the adult, but the adult may still transmit messages to the child. Messages of care, recognition, and proximity may be transmitted through the physical and vocal contact of the adult, even though the child with profound difficulties cannot understand these messages in the way that a more responsive person would.

Once children have shown some interest in the world and have begun responding to it, they are at Stage 2 of our scheme. Children who are at Stage 2 do not yet use speech, nor do they seem to understand it, but they are often lively and interested. Earlier it was noted that pre-verbal children will use actions such as tugging, crying, and so on, to convey messages for which speech will be used when they begin to talk. In this manual we have tried to bring some order to the range of actions which may be observed in the behaviour of children who are young developmentally. The system chosen is that which Piaget used to describe behaviour at the sensorimotor stage. These actions are listed in table 3 with explanations of their technical terms.

Through teaching activities based on these actions, pupils at Stage 2 will have opportunities to explore, manipulate, understand their surroundings, and notice details, and thus have a wide range of experiences which they may later express in words instead of actions and non-verbal vocalizations.

We acknowledge that this is but one way of classifying the activity of early childhood, and that other schemes are equally valid. For instance, a classification of purposeful behaviour could be derived from psycholinguistic sources such as Barrett (1980), Dale (1980), Dore (1975), or Halliday (1975). And Trevarthen's classification of the interpersonal behaviour of mothers and infants (1977) also has a powerful claim on the basis that it does credit to the complexity of communication, and gives priority to the interpersonal quality of communication rather than to the cognitive aspects which have been chosen here.

There are two striking characteristics of children at Stage 3. The first is that they show signs of understanding the language of other people. The second is that they begin to imitate this language. Imitation is a dramatic intimation of

Table 3 The six sensorimotor actions identified by Piaget

Action	Piagetian label	Explanation
1	The development of visual pursuit and the permanence of objects	Tracking moving objects; realizing that an object continues to exist after it has disappeared from view
2	The development of means for obtaining desired environmental events	Recognizing own power to change one's surroundings and meet one's own needs
3	The development of imitation: vocal and gestural	(Self-explanatory)
4	The development of operational causality	Recognizing cause–effect relationships
5	The construction of object relations in space	Realizing the importance of gravity, balance, and the position of objects in relation to each other
6	The development of schemes for relating to objects	Manipulating and exploring the properties of objects and materials (the naming of objects is the highest point on this scale)

(After Piaget 1936, 1937; Uzgiris and Hunt 1975)

growth in children's ability to communicate, even if adults are unable to find meaning in what the child has said. Imitation may have little communicative purpose as, for example, when it occurs in children who have autistic difficulties, and it is not particularly good as a predictor of later ability to communicate (Snyder 1975). This has not prevented sterile exercises in imitation becoming a dominant feature of many teaching schemes at the expense of activities based on the essentially purposeful and spontaneous nature of communication (Bryen and Joyce 1985).

The understanding of words is the ability which we should like to see developing at Stage 3 so that the pupils may begin to build up a bank of verbal concepts which will give them increased access to the broader communicative community. In fact, we shall see in the next section of the manual that 'Does the child understand any words?' is a key question to answer when deciding on an appropriate choice of activities for teaching at any point in the scheme.

Children's first words appear at Stage 4. These words may be conventional adult words, distorted conventional words, or words which the children themselves have invented. So long as they are recognized as referring consistently to particular objects, people, actions, feelings, positions, and so on, they are entitled to be called 'words'. The purpose of communication at Stage 4 is to use these first words to express feelings, to intimate wishes, to catch attention, and so on. You will find in Part 3 of the manual that some order has been brought to the task of classifying single words by dividing them into categories of function including commands, expression of wants and needs, and relating experiences, though we also give advice on eliciting words which you think the pupils may know, but do not use.

Stage 5 is the stage of connected speech, when children begin to combine words to form their first sentences, such as 'Mummy push', 'sit chair', and 'milk all gone'. This stage was created here, for practical and theoretical reasons. The practical reason was that, during our preparatory fieldwork, teachers often asked for advice on how to encourage children who could speak in single words to use connected speech. Therefore Stage 5 is in part a response to consumer demand. The theoretical reason for having the fifth stage is that two-word speech is different qualitatively from single-word speech. Some writers explain this by saying that the difference arises because children at the two-word stage have learned (1) that words may be linked, (2) that two or more ideas are related, and (3) how to express the relationship of these ideas in speech. Other writers prefer to explain the difference by saying that children at the two-word stage have overcome constraints such as inefficient immediate memory and processing of ideas. Readers who are interested in finding more about this debate will find that it has been summarized lucidly by Tager-Flusberg (1985).

The preceding discussion has explained the derivation of the five stages which act as a framework for teaching activities in Part 3 of the manual. Table 4 summarizes these stages and the principal aims for the teaching of communication at each of them.

Table 4 General teaching aims for the five stages

Stage	Description	Targets for activities
1	Children with profound learning difficulties	Make them aware of: sights sounds taste and smell touch movement
2	Children who have begun to take an active interest in their surroundings	Develop skills of thinking and action, such as: awareness of cause and effect awareness of position awareness of connections Develop recognition of sounds
3	Children who understand some words; children who have begun to imitate words	Help them to find meaning in words and other symbols Help them to imitate actions and sounds
4	Children who speak single words	Encourage them to produce words they understand Help them to realize that language is a useful tool
5	Children who use connected speech	Encourage them to produce more connected speech more often Extend their understanding of language Let them use language for a wider range of purposes

Using table 4 as a guide, it is not difficult to find teaching activities which are appropriate to each of the five stages. Table 5 provides some guidance on the kinds of activity which would suit the targets of table 4, and many more specific examples will be found in Part 3 of the manual. However, we hope that the guide will also help teachers devise, by their own ingenuity, appropriate activities for the children with whom they are working.

We should also add a word of caution. Communication is a very complex topic which cannot really be packaged into neat boxes such as those in table 5. Thus, the table should be useful as a general guide, but it should not make teachers feel restricted when they are planning work for their pupils. The boundaries of stages of development are not absolute; this is recognized both in developmental

Table 5 Relating the five stages to teaching activities

Stage	Description	Targets for activities	What to do
1	Children with profound learning difficulties	Make them aware of: sights sounds taste and smell touch movement	Find stimulation activities for each sense
2	Children who have begun to take an active interest in their surroundings	Develop skills of thinking and action, such as: awareness of cause and effect awareness of position awareness of connections Develop recognition of sounds	Find activities which encourage the child to reach, find things, watch things, make things happen, connect objects, use balance and gravity, respond to sounds (vocal, musical, instrumental)
3	Children who under-stand some words; children who have begun to imitate words	Help them to find meaning in words and other symbols Help them to imitate actions and sounds	Find activities which encourage the child to copy actions, copy sounds, take part in early make-believe play, attend to words
4	Children who speak single words	Encourage them to produce words they understand Help them to realize that language is a useful tool	Set up situations which encourage the child to produce words spontaneously. Avoid questions (especially those with yes/no answers) and demands if possible
5	Children who use connected speech	Encourage them to pro-duce more connected speech more often Extend their understand-ing of language Let them use language for a wider range of purposes	Find activities which help the child to: transmit information in a variety of ways broaden existing concepts

psychology (Piaget 1969) and in the practice of assessing and planning for children with severe learning difficulties (McConkey 1984). We crossed the boundaries of the five stages quite regularly when writing the teaching activities of Part 3. We hope that you will do the same.

Using *Early communicative skills*

The manual is not to be read from cover to cover. It was written as a teacher's handbook with information which could be consulted quickly in the course of daily practice or in preparation for it. The greater part of the manual therefore consists of a large collection of self-contained units, each of which is between one and three pages in length. The units are written in note-form, under a set of standard headings to make the information as accessible as possible to the reader (Horn, Nicol, Kleinmann, and Grace 1969). The units are grouped within three main sections dealing with:

- identification of each of the five stages of communication (Part 1 – pp. 13–24).
- activities for teaching (Part 2 – pp. 25–243).
- problems which teachers often encounter when working with children who have severe difficulties with communication (Part 3 – pp. 245–77).

It is important to recognize that these three sections are closely related; they are different points of focus on the same set of issues. For this reason, you will discover that there is extensive cross-referencing of units within and among the sections of the manual.

No single page is the right starting-point for every user of *Early communicative skills*. However, we suggest that you should consider beginning at one of the following three places if you are using the manual for the first time.

P. 13 if you want to discover what stage of communication the child you are working with has reached P. 13 lists the five stages of communication which are covered by *Early communicative skills*. Select the stage which seems to fit the child most closely, then read the pages which give details about that stage.

If you have any difficulty in selecting the most suitable stage, look again at table 2 (p. 5) and its supporting text.

Some children may seem to suit more than one stage. If this happens, select the most useful information from each stage's set of notes.

P. 25 if you are looking for a particular type of teaching activity P. 25 lists twenty groups of activities for helping children to communicate. These activities form the largest section of the book, that is, from page 27 to 242. Whenever possible, the less difficult activities in a group appear before the harder ones.

P. 245 if you are concerned about certain problems which prevent a child from communicating effectively Page 245 lists a selection of problems which are encountered quite frequently.

You will soon discover that *Early communicative skills* has a definite structure. One set of ideas is connected to several others in different parts of the manual. This structure will help you to build up a clearer picture of a child's ability and how to develop it.

Only one last point needs to be made about using the manual. Do not feel that you must follow its advice to the letter. Communication is too complex and people are too individual for any single book to have an answer to every single problem of teaching. Trust your own judgement. Adapt any activity to suit your needs. Question any opinion in the light of your experience.

What? No assessment charts?

Many sorts of assessment charts are used regularly in the schools. Some, like the PIP (Jeffree and McConkey 1976b) and the PAC (Gunzberg 1966), are published commercially; others are produced more informally. These charts can be useful for establishing the level at which a child is communicating; for judging if the child is making progress; and for suggesting new directions for work with the child. However, you will find no assessment charts in *Early communicative skills*. There are two main reasons for this.

The first is that we do not want to add unnecessarily to the range of charts used in the schools just now. The work in *Early communicative skills* can be related quite easily to any charts of communication which you are using already. Why create more paperwork?

The second reason is that communication is much too complex to be packaged into neat series of charted steps which are the same for all children. A really thorough assessment would be difficult to carry out and would take a long time. This time would be better spent working with the pupils, evaluating their needs and strengths, and discovering the circumstances in which they give of their best.

Early communicative skills will help you to assess and teach without making use of any special charts. You will be able to assess the child's level of communication by reading:

- What is communication at Stage 1 (2, 3, 4, or 5?)   pp. 15–24
- How else does the child appear at Stage 1 (2, 3, 4, or 5?) pp. 15–24
- Confusing cases   pp. 15–24

And you will be able to plan schemes of work for children by reading:

- Aims of work at Stage 1 (2, 3, 4, or 5)   pp. 15–24
- Types of work at Stage 1 (2, 3, 4, or 5)   pp. 15–24

- Moving on   pp. 15–24
- Moving on   pp. 25–242
- Less difficult activities   pp. 25–242

Keep records of the work you carry out. You may decide to use a note-book to act as an individual diary for each child. On the other hand, you may find it more useful to use a system of record-forms. There are some examples of simple forms between pp. 279 and 288. You may find them helpful if you wish to devise forms which are appropriate to your own needs.

Diary notes and record-forms, however informal, will often be an invaluable source of ideas on which to base the education of individual children.

Part 1

The development of communication

Stages in the development of communication

Stage 1: The children have profound learning difficulties   15

Stage 2: The children begin to take an active interest in their surroundings   17

Stage 3: The children begin to understand words and gestures   19

Stage 4: The children produce their own first words   21

Stage 5: The children use connected speech   23

Stage 1
The children have profound learning difficulties

KEY IDEAS

Stage 1 children have the most severe handicaps.
They are unresponsive.
They usually have severe physical handicaps as well as severe learning difficulties.

WHAT IS COMMUNICATION AT STAGE 1?

The children make no attempt to communicate.
Only rarely do the children try to reach out to the world round about them.
Adults try to communicate with the children by stimulating them.

HOW ELSE MAY THE PUPILS APPEAR AT STAGE 1?

They may smile when people talk to them or stroke them — but this is probably a reflex act only.
They may kick or move their limbs if their position of lying is changed — this may also just be reflex.
They may suck or mouth though there is no food near them.
They may make vocal sounds for no apparent reason.

CONFUSING CASES

Extremely withdrawn children   They are unresponsive and do not want to communicate. Almost every one of them will be above Stage 1.
   Go to Stage 3, p. 19, at least, if you think that a child can understand words.
   Go to Stage 2, p. 17, if they do not seem to understand words.
   Use plenty of non-verbal activities even if you think you are never going to encourage them to speak. Try to organize some system or timetable into their school day. There is good advice about organization and timetabling in *Teaching Children with Severe Behaviour/Communication Disorders* (Van Witsen 1977).
   See p. 267 of the manual for some general advice.

Severely physically handicapped children   The learning difficulties of these children may seem greater than they really are.

Go to Stage 2 (at least) if you are working with a child who
● enjoys company.
● likes or dislikes certain people.
● gets excited when something pleasant is going to happen.

AIMS OF WORK AT STAGE 1

To stimulate the sense of hearing (activities: pp. 27–40).
To stimulate the sense of vision (activities: pp. 41–8).
To stimulate the sense of touch (activities: pp. 49–56).
To stimulate the sense of movement (activities: pp. 57–66).
To stimulate the senses of taste and smell (activities: pp. 67–76).
To discover any areas of thinking or experience which can be developed more directly at Stage 2 level (activities: pp. 77–150).

TYPES OF WORK

Activities which stimulate all the senses.

MOVING ON

Move on to Stage 2 if
● the children respond deliberately or purposefully when you stimulate them.
● the children are taking an interest in their surroundings.
● the children recognize familiar people.

Stage 2
The children begin to take an active interest in their surroundings

KEY IDEAS

The children find out that they can influence people and manipulate objects.
They do not understand language.

WHAT IS COMMUNICATION AT STAGE 2?

Enjoyment of people's company.
Recognition of familiar people.
Attracting attention by use of the voice (though no words are used).
Reaching out towards people to attract attention.

HOW ELSE MAY THE PUPILS APPEAR AT STAGE 2?

They are mobile.
They follow moving objects with their gaze (if they can see).
They reach out for things.
They recognize familiar people.
They take an interest in their surroundings.
They examine objects.
They turn towards unexpected sounds.
They seem to recognize certain sounds, perhaps a voice, or a special toy, or a
    particular kind of music.
They play by hitting, patting, or shaking objects.

CONFUSING CASES

Extremely withdrawn children They are unresponsive and do not want to
communicate (so it seems). Go to Stage 3, at least, if you think that a child can
understand words. Use plenty of non-verbal activities, and try to introduce some
system or timetable into the child's school day.

There is good advice about organization and timetabling in *Teaching Children
with Severe Behaviour/Communication Disorders* (Van Witsen 1977).

The most profoundly handicapped children Some of these children look more
advanced than they really are. They may smile if talked to, or if they are stroked.

They may appear to explore toys or the surfaces that they are lying on. If Stage 2 work turns out to be unsuccessful, maybe it is because the children's behaviour is less purposeful than it seems. Try Stage 1 instead. See p. 15.

AIMS OF WORK AT STAGE 2

To increase awareness of sounds.
To increase powers of thinking.
To develop relationships with other people.

TYPES OF WORK AT STAGE 2

Recognition and understanding of sounds (activities: pp. 141–54).
Watching and findings things (activities: pp. 77–86).
Purposeful behaviour (activities: pp. 109–20).
Making things happen (activities: pp. 121–30).
The positioning of objects (activities: pp. 131–40).
Handling objects (activities: pp. 87–108).
Imitation of actions and sounds (activities: pp. 155–67).

MOVING ON

Move on to Stage 3 work if
- the children frequently call for your attention by using their voice or by tugging at your clothes.
- the work suggested for Stage 2 seems too easy.
- the children understand some simple words — but make sure that they are following the words and not gestures or pointing or changes in your tone of voice.
- the children have copied actions or vocal sounds from another child or an adult.
- the children take part in make-believe play.

Stage 3
The children begin to understand words and gestures

KEY IDEAS

Understanding of adult language appears.
The children's own speech is not used yet, but they sometimes imitate the speech
  of other people.

WHAT IS COMMUNICATION AT STAGE 3?

The children recognize meaning in the words and gestures of other people.
The children's play shows that they have been watching and listening to other
  people.

HOW ELSE MAY THE PUPIL APPEAR AT STAGE 3?

They look round or stop what they are doing when they hear their name
  mentioned.
They get excited, or show some other sign of recognition, when a familiar word is
  spoken.
They wave 'bye-bye' in imitation of an adult's waving.
They try to join in simple games such as 'pat-a-cake' or 'round and round the
  garden'.

CONFUSING CASES

Echolalic children   These children imitate speech, so they may be at Stage 3.
They may also be beyond it. Make a word-record (see p. 283 for details). If any
real speech appears, go to Stage 4 or Stage 5. For some advice on dealing with
echolalia, see p. 275.

Children who appear to understand more language than they really do   This
may happen when they are really responding to the rise and fall of the adult's
speech. They also take a lot of meaning from the body-movements and mime
which most people use unconsciously. Body-movement, mime, and the rise
and fall of speech are all important types of real communication. However,
they can draw attention away from speech. Go to Stage 2 activities for developing listening if the child does not cope with the comprehension activities of
Stage 3.

Children who speak, but only rarely They may be silent because of a physical handicap. Check with the speech therapist, audiologist, and school doctor.

If there is a physical problem, a non-verbal system of language is worth trying (pp. 238–42). If there is no obvious physical problem, go to Stage 4 and experiment with the suggestions there. If they are too hard, return to Stage 3. Ask the school's psychologist about techniques for encouraging children to be more responsive. See pp. 263–70.

AIMS OF WORK AT STAGE 3

To enable children to understand words.
To encourage children to imitate actions and vocal sounds of their own accord.
To build up the range of vocal sounds which children will produce.

TYPES OF WORK AT STAGE 3

Bringing words to the child's notice (activities: pp. 176–89).
Early make-believe (activities: pp. 168–71).
Imitation of actions (visible) (activities: pp. 155–8).
Imitation of actions (invisible) (activities: pp. 159–63).
Production of a range of sounds (activities: pp. 164–7).

MOVING ON

Move on to Stage 4 if
● children produce the occasional word of their own accord.
● children understand quite a lot of speech without pointing and mime.
● children imitate a range of vocal sounds such as animal noises, vehicle noises, and, possibly, words.
● children use a range of vocal sounds during free play.

Stage 4
The children produce their own first words

KEY IDEAS

The children make specific sounds or hand-signs which carry specific meaning.

WHAT IS COMMUNICATION AT STAGE 4?

The children make themselves understood by means of words, hand-signs, or (perhaps) pointing at pictures or line-drawings.
These first words may not be the same as correct adult words (see p. 263).
The words show that the children

- can identify objects and people.
- are aware of objects and actions.
- notice differences in objects, people, and actions.
- can build relationships with people.

HOW ELSE MAY THE PUPILS APPEAR AT STAGE 4?

They can follow simple directions such as 'Wave bye-bye'.
They will point to some objects or people when asked to.
They will listen to short stories about a picture or toy.

CONFUSING CASES

Children who seem to understand a lot of language but do not speak Discover if they are really responding to the rise and fall of adult speech and not to the words. Discover if they are really responding to pointing or mime. If either of these is the case, try activities for Stage 3.

Discover if there is any physical barrier to speech. The school doctor, the speech therapist, and/or the audiologist will advise you. If there is a physical problem, a non-verbal system of communication is worth considering (see pp. 238–42). If there is no physical problem, persevere at Stage 4 or even try some of the comprehension exercises of Stage 5. If this is too hard, return to Stage 3.

Ask the school's psychologist for advice on techniques for encouraging children to be more responsive. See pp. 263–70 also.

Children who have spoken just the occasional word   Stage 4 work is suitable. So is some of the Stage 3 work on comprehension.

Children who make up their own words   Stage 4 work is suitable if their own words can usually be understood.

Children who use correct adult words, but not with the usual adult meaning   Many adults do this too. Stage 4 work is suitable.

Children who produce two-word utterances (e.g. 'my dog') which do not sound like proper two-word sentences, (e.g. 'kick ball')   See p. 265. Stage 5 work may be suitable, but change to Stage 4 if it is too difficult.

Echolalic children   Make a word-record; see p. 283 for details. Stage 5 is suitable if real connected speech appears. Stay at Stage 4 if the only real speech being *used* comes as single words. Stage 3 may be high enough for comprehension exercises if no real speech is *used*. To deal with echolalia, see p. 275.

AIMS OF WORK AT STAGE 4

To draw out spoken (or signed) words during teaching.
To encourage spontaneous use of words.
To extend the child's comprehension of words.

TYPES OF WORK AT STAGE 4

Encourage the child to use speech (activities: pp. 191–4).
Language acting as a tool (activities: pp. 195–211).
Understanding words which belong within certain useful categories (activities: pp. 212–17).

MOVING ON

Move on to Stage 5 if
● children use connected speech frequently.
● children can use a lot (20 to 50) of single words.
● the comprehension exercises of Stage 4 are too easy.

Stage 5
The children use connected speech

KEY IDEA

The children combine words to make their meaning more clear.

WHAT IS COMMUNICATION AT STAGE 5?

Speech is used to control other people, to give information, and to work things out.
The meanings of many new words are learned.
Older words are learned more thoroughly.

HOW ELSE MAY THE PUPILS APPEAR AT STAGE 5?

They can follow more complicated commands than those at Stage 4 (e.g. they
can follow 'Bring an apple', or 'Get your gloves').
They can imitate new words easily.
They use language (perhaps just single words) to ask for things they want.
They recognize some objects and people in pictures and photographs.
They enjoy pretend play (e.g. putting a doll to bed, feeding a Teddy bear).
They 'help' an adult to get them dressed.

CONFUSING CASES

Echolalic children Make a word-record (see p. 283 for details). Go to Stage
4 if the only real speech (that is, speech which is used for a purpose) is the
occasional single word. Stay at Stage 5 if you record a lot of single words
or even connected speech being used. If no real speech is being used, Stage 3
may make sense. For advice on dealing with echolalia, see p. 275.

*Children who produce two-word utterances (e.g. 'my dog') which do not sound
like proper two-word sentences (e.g. 'kick ball')* Stage 5 work may be suitable,
but change to Stage 4 if it is too difficult.

Children who seem to understand a lot of language but do not speak Discover
if they are really responding to the rise and fall of adult speech and not to
the actual words. Discover if they are responding to pointing or mime. If
either of these is the case, you may have to look at the work for Stage 3.

Discover if there is any physical reason that the child does not speak. The
school doctor, speech therapist, or audiologist will advise you. Consider using

a non-verbal system of language (see pp. 238–42) if there is a physical problem.

If there is no physical problem, persevere with the exercises of Stage 4 and Stage 5. Ask the school's psychologist about techniques for encouraging children to be more responsive. See pp. 263–70 also.

AIMS OF WORK AT STAGE 5

To draw out connected speech during teaching.
To encourage spontaneous use of connected speech.
To extend the child's comprehension of words and concepts.

TYPES OF WORK AT STAGE 5

Drawing out connected speech by formal teaching (activities: pp. 225–8).
Drawing out connected speech by informal teaching (activities: pp. 229–31).
Developing the uses to which speech is put (activities: pp. 232–7).
Increasing understanding of the complexity of language (activities: pp. 212–20).
Increasing understanding of simple concepts (activities: pp. 221–4).

MOVING ON

Move on from Stage 5 if
● the children use connected speech as often as they use single words.
● the most advanced comprehension exercises in this manual are too easy.
See p. 243 for sources of ideas for work in communication beyond Stage 5.

Part 2

Activities for developing communication

Activities

Stimulating hearing   27
Stimulating vision   41
Stimulating the sense of touch   49
Stimulating the sense of movement   57
Stimulating the sense of smell   67
Stimulating the sense of taste   75
Watching and finding things   77
Handling objects   87
Behaving purposefully   109
Making things happen   121
Understanding the positioning of objects   131
Recognizing and understanding sounds   141
Imitating actions   155
Imitating vocal sounds   164
Make-believe play   168
Understanding words   176
Producing first words   191
More advanced understanding of language   212
Producing more advanced language   225
Language without speech   238

Beyond two-word sentences   243

Stimulating hearing and vision
Dangling toys

AIM

To let children experience a range of sounds.
To encourage children to produce sounds by touching objects.

SUITABILITY

The activity is suitable for
- the most profoundly handicapped children.
- children who are blind.
- children who are at Stage 1 (p. 150) of our scheme for the development of communication.

MATERIALS

Small toys which can be suspended on strings and which will sound easily when touched or struck.
Commercially produced rattles and bells.
Home-made items such as plastic containers holding some dried peas, rice, or barley.
A cross-bar for attaching the suspending strings. A broom-handle can be laid across the sides of a cot. Small 'goal-posts' will be needed for children lying on the floor or in wheelchairs.
Instead of cross bar/goal-posts, attach suspending strings to hooks in the ceiling, or attach two corners of a net to the ceiling and the other two to a wall. Tie strings for the toys to any part of the net.

PROCEDURE

(a) With the most profoundly handicapped children, *you* will have to make the toys sound. Short spells of five minutes will be sufficient.
(b) If the children can move their limbs, hang the toys where they have the best chance of striking them accidentally.
(c) Also try attaching an elastic cord from the toy to the children's wrist or ankle so that they are likely to produce a sound if they move.

TEACHING HINTS

1 Five to ten minutes will be long enough to spend on this activity at any one time.

27

2 Don't let 'accidental activities' such as (b) and (c) take the place of the real one-to-one work in (a).
3 Are there any sounds or movements in the room which may be distracting the children's attention? Try to cut them out when you want to keep the children's attention directed at one particular activity.
4 If possible, put away the toys when they are not in use. The children may notice them less and less if they are nearby all the time.

RECORD-KEEPING

Use a diary to keep note of any interesting reactions.

MOVING ON

Move on if the children
• are clearly interested in what is going on (they may smile, gurgle, move about, or turn towards you).
• seem to be reaching for the dangling toys.
• seem to be trying deliberately to make the dangling toys sound.

Look at activities for developing recognition of sounds (pp. 141–54). Look also at the activities which appear between pp. 74 and 140. Pages 77, 87, 109, 121, or 131 would be good starting-points.

LESS DIFFICULT ACTIVITIES

This activity is at the lower end of the range covered by the *Early Communicative Skills*. The remainder of the activities in this section are between pp. 29 and 76.

See also Jeffree and McConkey (1976a), Jeffree, McConkey, and Hewson (1977a), and Stevens (1976).

Stimulating hearing
Percussion and other simple instruments

AIM

To let the children hear a wide range of sounds.

SUITABILITY

The activity is suitable for
- the most profoundly handicapped children.
- children who are at Stage 1 (p. 15) of our scheme for the development of communication.

MATERIALS

Commercially-produced sounding toys: bells, rattles, cymbals, tambourines, drums, whistles.

Home-made toys: plastic containers or cocoa tins holding some barley, rice, dried peas, gravel, or a marble, empty tins (to be used as drums).

PROCEDURE

Produce the sounds in as many ways as possible — loudly or quietly, drawn-out or short, randomly or rhythmically, raspingly or smoothly. Pitch and tone-quality will vary from one instrument to the next.

Five minutes at a time will be long enough for this activity.

TEACHING HINTS

1 Talk to, and smile at the children, especially if they respond in any way.
2 Are there any sounds or movements in the room which may distract the children?
3 Do the children have any special likes or dislikes among the sounds you are making?

RECORD-KEEPING

Use a diary to keep note of any interesting reactions.

MOVING ON

Move on if children reach out for any of your sound-making toys, become excited, or show interest in what you are doing.

Look at the activities which appear between pp. 77 and 140. Pages 77, 87, 109, 121, or 131 would be good starting points.

Look also at activities for developing recognition of sounds (pp. 141–54).

LESS DIFFICULT ACTIVITIES

This activity is at the lower end of the range covered by *Early Communicative Skills*. The remainder of the activities in this section are between pages 27 and 76.

See also Jeffree and McConkey (1976a), Jeffree, McConkey, and Hewson (1977a), and Stevens (1976).

Stimulating hearing
Live music

AIM

To let children hear a wide range of sounds.

SUITABILITY

The activity is suitable for
- the most profoundly handicapped children. Also suitable for any other children, as a recreational activity.
- children from the level of Stage 1 (p. 15) of our scheme for the development of communication.

MATERIALS

Any musical instrument.

PROCEDURE

If you can play a musical instrument, or even make it sound, let the children hear it occasionally.

TEACHING HINTS

1 Five to ten minutes at a time will be long enough for this activity.
2 Note any response the children make when you play.
3 Note any response the children make when you stop.
4 Are there any sounds or movements in the room which may distract attention? Try to cut them out when you want the children to pay attention to certain specific sounds.

RECORD-KEEPING

Use a diary to keep note of any interesting reactions.

MOVING ON

Move on to activities for developing recognition of sounds (pp. 141–54), if the children respond noticeably when you play.

Look at the activities between pp. 77 and 140 if the children reach to touch the instrument. The activities on pp. 77, 87, 109, 121, or 131 would be good starting-points.

LESS DIFFICULT ACTIVITIES

This activity is at the lower end of the range covered by *Early Communicative Skills*. The remainder of the activities in this section are between pp. 27 and 76.

See also Jeffree and McConkey (1976a), Jeffree, McConkey, and Hewson (1977a), and Stevens (1976).

Stimulating hearing
Nursery rhymes and songs

AIM

To draw children's attention to the sounds of language.

SUITABILITY

The activity is suitable for
• the most profoundly handicapped children.
• children who are at Stage 1 (p. 15) of our scheme for the development of communication.

MATERIALS

None, or any book of well-known nursery rhymes (e.g. the Ladybird 822 series).

PROCEDURE

Hold the child in your arms, or sit or kneel nearby. Speak, read, or sing, taking any opportunity to emphasize rhythm, or changes in the tone of your voice.

Some children may be able to look at the book (if you are reading), but they will not pick out any details in the pictures. Therefore, do not spend time trying to direct their attention to the pictures unless you have a particularly good reason.

TEACHING HINTS

1 Children with profound learning difficulties will not be able to supply words that you deliberately miss out at the end of lines. This comes much later (see p. 193).
2 Five to ten minutes at a time will be long enough for this activity.
3 Talk to, and smile at the children, especially if they respond in any way.
4 Are there any sounds or movements in the room which will distract attention?
5 Note any rhymes or songs which the children respond to strongly.

RECORD-KEEPING

Use a diary or day-sheet to keep note of any interesting reactions.

MOVING ON

Move on to activities for developing recognition of sounds (pp.141–54) if the children show any interest or excitement when you are talking or singing.

LESS DIFFICULT ACTIVITIES

This activity is at the lower end of the range covered by *Early Communicative Skills*. The remainder of the activities in this section are between pp. 27 and 76.

See also Jeffree and McConkey (1976a), Jeffree, McConkey, and Hewson (1977a), and Stevens (1976).

Stimulating hearing
Background musical sounds

AIM

To let the children hear a wide range of sounds, without any direct supervision by an adult.

SUITABILITY

The activity is suitable for
- the most profoundly handicapped children.
- children who are at Stage 1 (p. 15) of our scheme for the development of communication.

MATERIALS

Recorded music (gramophone or tape recorder), clockwork musical toys, bells activated by wind or heat.

PROCEDURE

Note if the children's attention is caught by any particular type of music. Ask their parents if you are not sure.

Tape-record perhaps a dozen different kinds of music and play them to the children. Are there any interesting effects? Do they respond differently to different types of music?

It is also possible to obtain Japanese bells and bamboo mobiles which make sounds if they hang in a current of air.

Musical tones like these can often be played to the children without any close supervision by an adult.

TEACHING HINTS

1 Don't let these sounds and music play continuously. If they do, the children may stop noticing them and the staff may be irritated by them.
2 Are there any unwanted background sounds which may distract the children's attention? Try to cut them out when you want them to pay attention to certain specific sounds.

RECORD-KEEPING

Use a diary to keep note of any interesting reactions.

MOVING ON

Move on to activities for developing recognition of sounds (pp. 141–54), if the children show interest or excitement when the sounds are being produced.

LESS DIFFICULT ACTIVITIES

This activity is at the lower end of the range covered by *Early Communicative Skills*. The remainder of the activities in this section are between pp. 27 and 76.

See also Jeffree and McConkey (1976a), Jeffree, McConkey, and Hewson (1977a), and Stevens (1976).

Stimulating senses of hearing and touch
Finger rhymes

AIM

To stimulate the sense of touch.

SUITABILITY

The activity is suitable for
• the most profoundly handicapped children.
• less handicapped children who have begun to explore the world.
• children at Stages 1 and 2 (pp. 15–18) of our scheme for the development of communication.

MATERIALS

None, or any nursery rhyme book which contains action rhymes — examples will be found among the Ladybird Nursery Rhymes Series (Series 822).

PROCEDURE

Seat the child on your knee, or sit side by side.
　　Read or recite any finger rhymes that you choose, going through the actions with the child.
　　Let your voice vary in pitch, rhythm, and intensity to make the sound of the activity interesting.

TEACHING HINTS

1　Five to ten minutes of this activity will be sufficient at any one time.
2　Note if the child responds strongly to any particular rhyme or activity.
3　The most profoundly handicapped children will not show any signs of anticipation just before an interesting part of the rhyme is spoken. A child who shrugs away or giggles *before* being tickled is showing anticipation and understanding. Make a note when you see it.

RECORD-KEEPING

Use a diary to keep note of any interesting reactions.

MOVING ON

Move on to some of the easier activities between pp. 77 and 140 if the children anticipate the exciting parts of a nursery rhyme. The activities on pp. 77, 87, 109, 121, and 131 could be good starting-points.

Look also at the most simple activities for developing recognition of sounds (pp. 141–54).

Continue to use finger rhymes as an activity — many children who can speak find it entertaining, and may overcome shyness to take part in it.

LESS DIFFICULT ACTIVITIES

This activity is at the lower end of the range covered by *Early Communicative Skills*. The remainder of the activities in this section are between pp. 27 and 76.

See also Jeffree, McConkey, and Hewson (1977a) and Stevens (1976).

Stimulating hearing and movement
Sounds from leg movement

AIM

To let children hear a range of sounds.
To make children aware that their legs exist.
To encourage deliberate movement of the legs.

SUITABILITY

The activity is suitable for
- the most profoundly handicapped children.
- children who are Stage 1 (p. 15) of our scheme for the development of communication.

MATERIALS

Sheets of brown paper, cellophane wrapping, or any other flexible, noisy material.

PROCEDURE

Check with a physiotherapist, nurse, or doctor that this activity is safe for the children.

Spread a sheet of paper under the children's feet on the cot or mattress. Gently drop one or both feet on to the paper so that it sounds.

Alternatively, hold the ankles and gently drum the feet and legs against the paper.

TEACHING HINTS

1 Five minutes at a time will be long enough for this activity.
2 Talk to, and smile at the children, especially if they respond in any way.
3 Are there any sounds or movements in the room which may distract the children?
4 You may decide to leave the paper in position when the children are lying unattended. This may encourage them to move. However, it may also cause loss of interest and you would then have to look around for some new, more interesting surface.

RECORD-KEEPING

Use a diary to keep note of any interesting reactions.

MOVING ON

Move on if the children seem to be moving their legs deliberately or if they are clearly interested in what is going on.

Look at the activities which appear between pp. 77 and 140. Pages 77, 87, 109, 121, and 131 would be good starting-points. Look also at activities for developing recognition of sounds (pp. 141–54).

LESS DIFFICULT ACTIVITIES

This activity is at the lower end of the range covered by *Early Communicative Skills*. The remainder of the activities in this section are between pp. 27 and 76.

See also Jeffree and McConkey (1976a), Jeffree, McConkey, and Hewson (1977a), and Stevens (1976).

Stimulating vision
Showing a variety of toys and household objects

AIM

To encourage focusing on objects.
Later, to encourage inspection of them.

SUITABILITY

The activity is suitable for
- the most profoundly handicapped children.
- children who are at Stage 1 (p. 15) of our scheme for the development of communication.
  The activity is not suitable for children with very severe visual impairment.

MATERIALS

Many toys or household objects. The size will depend on how you intend to use them.

PROCEDURE

(a) The children sit on your knee, or facing you in a wheelchair or other support. Try to direct the children's attention to the object by bringing it into their line of vision, or by moving their head so that their gaze is directed at it. Guide their hands over the object, if possible.
(b) Place medium-size objects such as spoons, dolls, or squeezy toys in the children's hands. Guide their hands around the object to discover any interesting properties such as sound or texture.

TEACHING HINTS

1 Ten minutes of this activity at a time should be sufficient.
2 Note if children respond markedly to any particular object.
3 Don't leave children lying with an object in their hands for a long time. This may make them lose any interest they had in it.
4 Are there any distracting sounds or movements in the room? Try to cut them out when you want to keep children's attention on one specific activity.
5 Talk to the children as you work with them to direct their attention, to keep up their interest, and to encourage voluntary action.

RECORD-KEEPING

Use a diary or day-sheet (p. 281) to keep note of any interesting reactions.

MOVING ON

Move on to the activities between pp. 77 and 108 if the children move their hands around an object or seem to be examining it.

Move to the activities between pp. 109 and 140 if they move their hands or gaze towards an object which has fallen or is out of reach.

LESS DIFFICULT ACTIVITIES

This activity is at the lower end of the range covered by *Early Communicative Skills*. The remainder of the activities in this section are between pp. 27 and 76.

See also Jeffree, McConkey, and Hewson (1977a) and Stevens (1976).

Stimulating vision
Displays of movement

AIM

To catch the children's attention.
To encourage the development of eye movement.

SUITABILITY

The activity is suitable for
- the most profoundly handicapped children.
- children who are at Stage 1 (p. 15) of our scheme for the development of communication.
  The activity is not suitable for children with very severe visual impairment.

MATERIALS

Mobiles, either home-made or commercially-produced.
Any toys which can be made to swing.
Mechanical and roll-along toys.
Paper darts and gliders.
A torch (its beam can be played on the ceiling).
Disco strobe-lighting or revolving lights.
Wax-filled lamp.

PROCEDURE

Set any of these objects in motion. Make sure that they are in the children's line of vision, and, if necessary, guide their head (with your hands) to the best possible position.

If the children do look at an object, gradually move it away from their gaze to see if they will follow it.

TEACHING HINTS

1 Five to ten minutes of this activity at a time will be sufficient.
2 Are there any distracting sounds or movements in the room? Try to cut them out when you want children's attention to be concentrated on one specific activity.
3 The children may not be able to follow much movement with their eyes. Do not rush to produce very noticeable eye-movement or head-movement to keep track of an object.

4 Note if the children respond markedly to any particular object.
5 Talk to the children to direct their attention, keep up their interest, and encourage any voluntary action.

RECORD-KEEPING

Use a diary or day-sheet (p. 281) to keep note of any interesting reactions.

MOVING ON

Move on to the activities between pp. 77 and 86 if you see the children beginning to track movement with their eyes.

Move on to the activities between pp. 109 and 120 if you see the children reaching out to touch the object.

LESS DIFFICULT ACTIVITIES

This activity is at the lower end of the range covered by *Early Communicative Skills*. The remainder of the activities in this section are between pp. 27 and 76.

See also Jeffree, McConkey, and Hewson (1977a) and Stevens (1976).

Stimulating vision
Real-life displays

AIM

To catch children's attention at times when staff are not working them.

SUITABILITY

The activity is suitable for
● the most profoundly handicapped children, if they have adequate vision.
● less handicapped children who are unable to move about to keep themselves amused.
● children who are at Stages 1 and 2 (pp. 15–18) of our scheme for the development of communication.

MATERIALS

Aquarium.
Window-seat (or mattress) with a view over the playground, so that other children can be seen moving around.
School animals in a pen.

PROCEDURE

Lay or seat the children once or twice a day in a position where they have a good chance of seeing what is happening in one or other of the displays mentioned above.

TEACHING HINTS

1 Background music is not noticed when we get too much of it. So is background visual stimulation. Do not let this activity take the place of all other work, unless the children are ill.
2 Alter seating position, direction of gaze, or the position of anything else which prevents the children from having a clear view of what you want them to see.
3 Encourage any interest the children show in what is going on.
4 Note if the children respond strongly to anything that they see or hear.

RECORD-KEEPING

Make occasional notes in the child's diary.

MOVING ON

Move on to the activities between pp. 77 and 86 if the children's gaze follows what is happening.

Move on to the activities between pp. 77 and 86 if they try to reach for anything.

Look also at activities for developing recognition of sounds — they begin on p. 141.

LESS DIFFICULT ACTIVITIES

This activity is at the lower end of the range covered by *Early Communicative Skills*. The remainder of the activities in this section are between pp. 27 and 76.

See also Jeffree, McConkey, and Hewson (1977a) and Stevens (1976).

Stimulating vision
The display wedge

AIM

To catch the children's attention, to encourage the development of eye-movement, and to encourage focusing on objects.

SUITABILITY

The activity is suitable for
- profoundly handicapped children with adequate vision.
- children who are at Stages 1 and 2 (pp. 15–18) of our scheme for the development of communication.

MATERIALS

Display wedge — details are provided in *Let Me Play*, p. 63 (Jeffree, McConkey, and Hewson 1977a).
Movable toys (balls, cars, small animals-on-wheels).

PROCEDURE

Check with a parent, doctor, nurse, or physiotherapist that it is safe for the children to lie face down.

Lay the children face down on the wedge. Decide on a comfortable position for their arms, and check that their view of the floor is not blocked.

Play with the moving toys within their line of vision. Talk to them and make animal (or vehicle) noises to catch their attention.

Note if they respond strongly to any of the sounds you are making. Tongue-clucking to imitate a horse's hooves is a good example.

Move the children's head to direct their attention, if necessary.

If you do not have a display wedge, the roller (p. 57) can be used instead.

TEACHING HINTS

1 Ten minutes of this activity at a time will be enough. Make it shorter if the children show signs of discomfort or distress.
2 Do they respond to any toys or sounds especially strongly? If so, keep these toys 'special' by using them just for teaching purposes or as rewards for extra effort.

3 Are there any distracting sounds or movements in the room? Try to cut out as many of these as possible from children's attention.
4 The children may not be able to follow much movement with their eyes. Do not rush to produce very noticeable eye-movements or head-movements to keep track of an object.
5 Show the children that they can reach for objects, but do not rush this.
6 Encourage any voluntary efforts by the children.

RECORD-KEEPING

Use a diary or day-sheet (p. 281).

MOVING ON

Move on to the activities between pp. 77 and 86 if the children follow moving objects with their eyes.

Move on to the activities between pp. 109 and 120 if the children appear to be reaching for any object.

Move on to activities for developing recognition of sounds (pp. 141–54) if the children seem to be interested in any sounds you make.

LESS DIFFICULT ACTIVITIES

This activity is at the lower end of the range covered by *Early Communicative Skills*. The remainder of the activities in this section are between pp. 27 and 76.

See also Jeffree and McConkey (1976a), Jeffree, McConkey, and Hewson (1977a) and Stevens (1976).

Stimulating the sense of touch
Differences in texture

AIM

To develop awareness of a variety of textures.

SUITABILITY

The activity is suitable for
- the most profoundly handicapped children.
- children who are at Stage 1 (p. 15) of our scheme for the development of communication.

MATERIALS

Hard things   spoons, building bricks, empty cocoa tins.
Objects with 'give' plastic cups, rubber balls, sponges.
Spiky objects   hairbrushes, toothbrushes, combs.
Rough surfaces   a variety of pot scourers, sandpaper.
Soft things   cotton-wool, flannel, paintbrushes.
Pliable things   crinkly paper from boxes of biscuits and chocolates, play-dough (the home-made kind which feels like putty).

PROCEDURE

Choose a variety of different textures, using the above list as a guide. Place the objects, one at a time, between the children's hands and press them together.

Sometimes (e.g. with sandpaper) it will be better to draw the children's hand across the surface of the object rather than squeeze it.

Some materials will be suitable to brush the children's face and the soles of their feet — this makes it an activity for developing body-image too.

TEACHING HINTS

1 Up to ten minutes at a time could be spent on this activity.
2 Take note of any textures to which the child responds strongly.
3 Encourage any voluntary action which the children make.
4 Finnie (1974) is not keen on special stimulation sessions using only small pieces of material. She prefers larger, interesting, everyday things which can be found around the house.

RECORD-KEEPING

Use a diary or day-sheet (p. 281).

MOVING ON

Move on to the activities between pages 77 and 140 if the children explore the materials in a deliberate fashion with their eyes, hands, or mouth. Pages 77, 87, 109, 121, or 131 might be good starting-points.

LESS DIFFICULT ACTIVITIES

This activity is at the lower end of the range covered by *Early Communicative Skills*. The remainder of the activities in this section are between pages 27 and 76.

See also Jeffree and McConkey (1976a), Jeffree, McConkey, and Hewson (1977a), and Stevens (1976).

Stimulating the sense of touch
Towelling

AIM

To increase the child's awareness of the sense of touch and, to some extent, of heat. To develop body-image.

SUITABILITY

This activity is suitable for
• the most profoundly handicapped children.
• physically handicapped children.
• children with poor body-image.
• children who are at Stages 1 and 2 (pp. 15–18) of our scheme for the development of communication.

MATERIALS

A bath or hand towel.
Mattress or comfortable spring matting.

PROCEDURE

Check with a parent, doctor, nurse, or physiotherapist that this activity will not injure the children.

Remove the children's outer clothes so that their arms and legs (at least) are exposed.

Beginning at the fingers, rub the towel along and around the arm as if you were drying the child very thoroughly.

Talk to the children about what you are doing, mentioning each of the parts of the arm along the way. A profoundly handicapped child will not understand what you are saying, but your voice will give additional human contact and experience of communication.

When you have towelled both arms, start on the legs, beginning with the toes.

TEACHING HINTS

1 The room temperature should be comfortable for the children.
2 Spend up to ten minutes on this activity at any one time. It could take place more than once a day if the child's timetable of activities is not full.

RECORD-KEEPING

Keep notes in a diary.

MOVING ON

Exploration, searching, reaching, and similar behaviour will occur if a child advances beyond the most profound degree of handicap. However, clumsier children may continue having exercises such as this one. Ask a physiotherapist for advice.

Read *Handling the Young Cerebral Palsied Child at Home* (Finnie 1974).

LESS DIFFICULT ACTIVITIES

This activity is at the lower end of the range covered by *Early Communicative Skills*. The remainder of the activities in this section are to be found between pages 27 and 76.

See also Jeffree and McConkey (1976a), Jeffree, McConkey, and Hewson (1977a) and Stevens (1976).

Stimulating the sense of touch and movement
Foot exercises

AIM

To let children experience a variety of skin sensations at their feet.
To enhance body-image.

SUITABILITY

The activity is suitable for
• the most profoundly handicapped children.
• children who are at Stage 1 (p. 15) of our scheme for the development of
  communication.

MATERIALS

Large basin, baby's bath, or wash-tub.
Expanded polystyrene chippings (packing for electrical goods).
Foam-sponge chippings (stuffing for pillows).
Sand.
Straw.
Warm water.

PROCEDURE

Take off the children's socks and shoes.
   Seat them with their feet in the tub (or bath) which can contain chippings,
straw, sand, warm water, or any other substance which you think could be
interesting.
   Move their feet around in the tub, talking about what you are doing. You can
say things such as 'Round and round we go' or 'Splish, splash' — this will add
more human contact to the physical contact of holding the ankles or feet.

TEACHING HINTS

1 Five minutes of this activity at any one time may be enough for you.
2 Note any substances to which the children respond strongly.
3 You can leave some children unattended during this activity, but that may make
  them lose interest in it.
4 Encourage any voluntary action.

RECORD-KEEPING

Use a diary or day-sheet (p. 281).

MOVING ON

Move on to the activities between pages 109 and 130 if children move their legs of their own accord in the tub.

Look also at the activities for developing recognition of sounds — they begin on p. 141.

The foot-movement activity may be worth keeping for recreation, even when the children have advanced beyond it.

LESS DIFFICULT ACTIVITIES

This activity is at the lower end of the range covered by *Early Communicative Skills*. The remainder of the activities in this section are between pages 27 and 76.

See also Jeffree, McConkey, and Hewson (1977a) and Stevens (1976).

Stimulating the sense of touch and movement
Foot-painting

AIM

To let children experience interesting sensations of touch and movement at
their feet.
To develop body-image.

SUITABILITY

The activity is suitable for
- the most profoundly handicapped children.
- children who have begun to explore the world.
- children who are at Stages 1 and 2 (pp. 15–18) of our scheme for the development of communication.

MATERIALS

Finger paints; alternatively, mix washing-up liquid with poster paints.
Painting board with plastic laminate surface.
Metal tray for holding paint.

PROCEDURE

Remove the children's socks and shoes.
　　Seat them at the board for foot-painting. If they are severely physically
handicapped you will need to use a chair which supports them from the back
and from the sides.
　　Make the children's feet slip about on the board. If they are attentive and if
they can see, show them the patterns their feet are making.

TEACHING HINTS

1　Five minutes of this activity may be enough at any one time.
2　This is an exercise in stimulation rather than creativity. Do not expect children
　　to move their feet of their own accord, but show them that you are pleased
　　if they do.
3　Talk to the children as you work with them and encourage any movements
　　they may make of their own accord.

RECORD-KEEPING

Use a diary or day-sheet (p. 281).

MOVING ON

Move on to the activities which appear between pp. 77 and 140 if chlidren move their feet of their own accord. Pages 77, 87, 109, 121, and 131 might be good starting-points.

However, retain foot-painting as a recreational activity if children enjoy it.

LESS DIFFICULT ACTIVITIES

This activity is at the lower end of the range covered by *Early Communicative Skills*. The remainder of the activities in this section are between pp. 27 and 76.

See also Jeffree, McConkey, and Hewson (1977a) and Stevens (1976).

Stimulating the sense of movement
The roller

AIM

To let children experience movement in prone position.
To let children experience the pull of gravity from different positions.
To give children the opportunity to look down on the world rather than up
at it.

SUITABILITY

The activity is suitable for
• the most profoundly handicapped children.
• some severely physically handicapped children.
• children with poor body-image.
• children who are at Stages 1 and 2 (pp. 15–18) of our scheme for the development of communication.

MATERIALS

A gymnastics mat, tightly rolled and tied, or a PVC roll from Totally Soft Play
Environment, or a home-made tubular bag made out of scrap material and stuffed
tightly with soft scrap materials (this could take the shape of a cylinder approximately 20 cm in diameter and 60 cm long).

PROCEDURE

**Check with a parent, doctor, nurse, or physiotherapist that this activity is
safe for the children.**

Lay the child across the roller with feet on one side and arms on the other.
    Hold the child by the thighs and gently push forward across the roller. Alter-
natively, lay the child astride the roller. Rock the child gently from side to side,
giving support at the hips or shoulders.
    If you do not have a display wedge (p. 47), the roller could be used instead
in that activity.

TEACHING HINTS

1 Look out for signs of distress or discomfort in the child. Stop if you see them.
2 Five minutes at a time will probably be enough to spend on this activity.

3 Note any responses the child makes during this activity.
4 Talk or sing to the child during the activity.
5 Give encouragement if the child seems to reach out for support when off balance
— for example, by stretching out to touch the ground.

RECORD-KEEPING

Use a diary or day-sheet.

MOVING ON

Move to the range of activities between pages 77 and 140 if the child regularly moves arms or legs purposefully when on the roller.

Continue to use this activity for exercise and recreation.

LESS DIFFICULT ACTIVITIES

This activity is at the lower end of the range covered by *Early Communicative Skills*. The remainder of the activities in this section are between pages 27 and 76.

See also Jeffree, McConkey, and Hewson (1977a) and Stevens (1976). Finnie (1974) gives good advice on working with severely physically-handicapped children.

Stimulating the sense of movement
Rocking-board

AIM

To make the children aware of the pull of gravity.
To encourage the children to react to the pull of gravity.

SUITABILITY

The activity is suitable for
• the most profoundly handicapped children.
• some severely physically handicapped children.
• children with poor body-image.
• children who are at Stages 1 and 2 (pp. 15–18) of our scheme for the development of communication.

MATERIALS

Home-made rocking board (see the drawing on next page).

PROCEDURE

Check with a parent, doctor, nurse, or physiotherapist that these activities are safe for the children.

If the children cannot stand, seat them (and support them) on the rocking-board. If you hold the sides of the board they can flop backwards against you for support if necessary.
    Rock the board from side to side.
    If the children can stand, support them standing on the board — hold their hands or the sides of the trunk to keep them steady.
    Rock the board from side to side as before.

TEACHING HINTS

1 Five minutes of this activity will be enough at any one time.
2 Stop if you see any signs of distress or discomfort.
3 Encourage any movement which seems to be aimed at keeping balance — for example, reaching with the arm to stop a sideways fall; bending and flexing legs in response to the movement.

RECORD-KEEPING

Use a diary or day-sheet (p. 281).

MOVING ON

Move on to the range of activities between pp. 77 and 140 if the children regularly use their arms or legs purposefully when they are on the board.

Continue to use this activity for exercise and recreation.

LESS DIFFICULT ACTIVITIES

This activity is at the lower end of the range covered by *Early Communicative Skills*. The remainder of the activities in this section are between pp. 27 and 76.

See also Jeffree, McConkey, and Hewson (1977a) and Stevens (1976). Finnie (1974) gives good advice on working with severely physically-handicapped children.

Illustration 1 Rocking-board

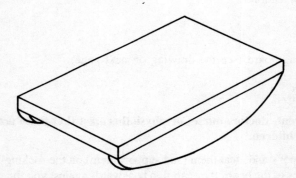

Seat is approximately 60 cm x 30 cm. Height from ground between 10 cm and 15 cm. Any strong wood or board could be used.

Stimulating the sense of movement
Angels in the snow

AIM

To develop awareness that the legs and arms can make large movements.

SUITABILITY

The activity is suitable for
• the most profoundly handicapped children.
• more able children with physical handicaps and with problems of body-image.
• children who are at Stages 1 and 2 (pp. 15–18) of our scheme for the development of communication.

MATERIALS

A large mat or mattress.

PROCEDURE

Check with a parent, doctor, nurse, or physiotherapist that this activity is safe for the children.

The children are laid on their back on the mat, legs as close together as possible, and arms by their sides.

   If the children are fairly small, kneel astride them and hold their hands and wrists. Bring their arms away from their sides, along the mat for as wide an arc of movement as is comfortable; if they have completely free movement their arms will end up above their head on the mat.

Look out for any signs of discomfort or distress. Stop and investigate if they appear.

If the children are too large for you to kneel astride their body, kneel astride the head, looking towards the feet. You then begin the exercise with a long stretch forward (for you!) to take the arms away from the sides.

   The leg exercise is less strenuous for you. Kneel at the children's feet. Take an ankle or foot in each hand and gently pull the legs away from each other along the mat.

TEACHING HINTS

1 Catch the children's gaze if possible. Smile and talk to them during this activity.
2 Encourage any voluntary attempts which they make at movement.
3 Remember that the leg's arc of movement is much less than the arm's. Imagine yourself in the child's position and you will bring the right degree of sympathy to the task.

RECORD-KEEPING

Keep notes in a diary.

MOVING ON

Move on if children seem to be making part of the movement of their own accord. Look at the range of non-verbal activities between pp. 77–140. Look also at the activities for developing recognition and understanding of sounds (pp. 141–54).

Finnie (1974) may give you some ideas for further physical activities with the child, but try to obtain first-hand advice from a physiotherapist.

LESS DIFFICULT ACTIVITIES

This activity is at the lower end of the range covered by *Early Communicative Skills*. The remainder of the activities in this section are to be found between pages 27 and 76.

See also Jeffree, McConkey, and Hewson (1977a) and Stevens (1976).

Stimulating the sense of movement
Swinging

AIM

To let children feel the range of movement and gravitational pull which occurs during swinging.

SUITABILITY

The activity is suitable for
• the most profoundly handicapped children.
• children who are at Stages 1 or 2 (pp. 15–18) of our scheme for the development of communication.

MATERIALS

None.

PROCEDURE

Check with a parent, doctor, nurse, or physiotherapist that this activity is safe for the children.
Do not attempt it if you are in any doubt about your own strength or fitness.

Hold the children in one of the following ways:
• facing them, hold them at the armpits.
• facing them, put your arms under their arms and clasp your hands behind their back.
• facing their back, hold them at their armpits.
• facing their back, pass your arms under theirs, and clasp your hands in front.
  Swing children gently at first. Bend and straighten your legs as you do it, to take the strain off your back.
  Talk to the children as you swing. Calling 'Wheee' will do, or you can say 'Up and down' in time with the movement.

TEACHING HINTS

1 Stop if you or the children experience discomfort or distress.
2 Thirty seconds of this activity can be very strenuous; ten may be enough at any one time.

3 Encourage any signs which suggest that children are enjoying themselves or are trying to take an active part.

4 Read pp. 47 and 50 of *Handling the Young Cerebral Palsied Child at Home* (Finnie 1974) for advice on spastic and athetoid children.

RECORD-KEEPING

Keep occasional notes in a diary.

MOVING ON

Move on to the range of activities between pp. 77 and 140 if you think children are trying to join in the activity with you. For example, they may hold out their hands to be lifted, or laugh or become more excited when you go to pick them up.

Continue to use this activity as a physical exercise and as recreation.

LESS DIFFICULT ACTIVITIES

This activity is at the lower end of the range covered by *Early Communicative Skills*. The remainder of the activities in this section are between pages 27 and 76.

See also Jeffree, McConkey, and Hewson (1977a) and Stevens (1976). Finnie (1974) gives good advice on working with severely physically-handicapped children.

Stimulating the sense of movement
Floor see-saw

AIM

To encourage arm-stretching and give exercise to the abdomen.

SUITABILITY

The activity is suitable for
• the most profoundly handicapped children.
• children at Stages 1 and 2 (pp. 15–18) of our scheme for the development of communication.
• as a game, or physical exercise, for most other children.

MATERIALS

A mattress, gymnastics mat, or any other floor-covering which will cushion the force of lowering the child's head and back to the floor.

PROCEDURE

Check with a parent, doctor, nurse, or physiotherapist that this activity is safe for the children.

Lay the children flat on their back.
 Kneel astride their legs somewhere between ankle and knee.
 Grasp the wrists, hands, or upper arms firmly.
 Pull them gently to a sitting position, then lower carefully. As you do this you can sing 'See saw, Marjory Daw', or simply say 'Up and down' or 'Hello, goodbye' in time with the movement.

TEACHING HINTS

1 Five minutes of this activity will be enough at any one time.
2 Stop if you see any signs of distress or discomfort.
3 Encourage any action of the children which suggests that they are trying to take an active part.

RECORD-KEEPING

Use a diary or day-sheet.

MOVING ON

Move on to the range of activities between pp. 77 and 140 if you are fairly sure that the child is trying to co-operate.

Continue to use this activity as a physical exercise and for recreation.

LESS DIFFICULT ACTIVITIES

This activity is at the lower end of the range covered by *Early Communicative Skills*. The remainder of the activities in this section are between pages 27 and 76.

See also Jeffree, McConkey, and Hewson (1977a) and Stevens (1976). Finnie (1974) gives good advice on working with severely physically handicapped children.

Stimulating the sense of smell
Smells around the house and school

AIM

To increase the range of smells which the children experience.

SUITABILITY

The activity is suitable for
- the most profoundly handicapped children.
- blind children.
- children who are at Stages 1 and 2 (pp. 15–18) of our scheme for the development of communication.

MATERIALS

None.

PROCEDURE

Let the children have experience of being in more than one room at home or school. Each room has its own smells because of the different activities which take place in it and because of furniture with a distinctive smell. For instance, the smell of a piano is unlike that of most other furniture.

Kitchens and home-economics rooms are also worth visiting. Profoundly handicapped children do not usually visit them because there is nothing they can take part in. Yet the smells there are often striking and pleasant, and he profoundly handicapped child in a wheelchair will cause few problems by being there.

TEACHING HINTS

Note if the children show a definite reaction to any particular smell. Talk to them about it.

RECORD-KEEPING

Use a diary to keep note of any interesting reactions.

MOVING ON

Children who take an interest in their surroundings are ready for some of the easier activities between pp. 77 and 140. The activities on pages 77, 87, 109, 121, and 131 could be suitable starting-points.

Look also at the most simple activities for developing recognition of sounds (pp. 141–54).

LESS DIFFICULT ACTIVITIES

This activity is at the lower end of the range covered by *Early Communicative Skills*. The remainder of the activities in this section are between pages 27 and 76.

See also Jeffree, McConkey, and Hewson (1977a) and Stevens (1976).

Stimulating the sense of smell
Smells from the open air

AIM

To increase the variety of smells which the children experience.

SUITABILITY

The activity is suitable for
• the most profoundly handicapped children.
• children with severe visual impairments.
• children at Stages 1 and 2 (p. 15–18) of our scheme for the development of communication.

MATERIALS

None.

PROCEDURE

Take the children into the open air as often as possible.

The fields, woods, and seaside provide many opportunities for experiencing interesting smells in rural areas. So do parks, shops, and factories in the bigger towns.

If there is no risk of hay-fever, children could lie on grass occasionally, and thus come closer to the smell of flowers and of the grass itself.

Your school may have a farm nearby. Take the children around the barns and pens to give them a change from indoor smells.

TEACHING HINTS

Talk to the children when you are on outings. This seems obvious advice, but it is more natural to talk to the other adults!

RECORD-KEEPING

Use a diary to keep note of any interesting reactions.

MOVING ON

Children who show an interest in their surroundings are ready for some of the easier activities between pp. 77 and 140. The activities on pp. 77, 87, 109, 121, and 131 could be suitable starting-points.

Look also at the most simple activities for developing recognition of sounds (pp. 141–54).

LESS DIFFICULT ACTIVITIES

This activity is at the lower end of the range covered by *Early Communicative Skills*. The remainder of the activities in this section are between pages 27 and 76.

See also Jeffree, McConkey, and Hewson (1977a) and Stevens (1976).

Stimulating the sense of smell
Perfumes and after-shaves

AIM

To increase the children's likelihood of identifying people.

SUITABILITY

The activity is suitable for
- the most profoundly handicapped children.
- children with severe visual impairments.
- children who are at Stages 1 and 2 of our scheme for the development of communication.

MATERIALS

Any perfume or after-shave, preferably not one which is shared by any of your colleagues.

PROCEDURE

Use a perfume or after-shave. This may have most educational advantage if you use only one, or if you restrict yourself to a small group, over the months.

When you meet children first thing in the morning, and when you go over to work with them, say 'Hello [their name] it's [your name] here', or something like that. This act of greeting, your voice, scent, and touch will mark you out even if the words are not understood.

TEACHING HINTS

Note if the children behave differently when they are with different members of staff.

RECORD-KEEPING

Use a diary to note any interesting reactions.

MOVING ON

Children who recognize certain people are ready for some of the easier activities between pp. 77 and 140. The activities on pages 77, 87, 109, 121, and 131 are suitable starting-points. Look also at the most simple activities for developing recognition of sounds (pp. 141–54).

LESS DIFFICULT ACTIVITIES

This activity is at the lower end of the range covered by *Early Communicative Skills*. The remainder of the activities in this section are between pages 27 and 76.

See also Jeffree, McConkey, and Hewson (1977a) and Stevens (1976).

Stimulating the sense of smell
Smells in boxes

AIM

To give experience of a range of smells.

SUITABILITY

The activity is suitable for
- the most profoundly handicapped children.
- children with severe visual impairment.
- non-verbal children who have begun to explore.
- children who are at Stages 1 and 2 (pp. 15–18) of our scheme for the development of communication.

MATERIALS

Empty boxes for Tic-Tac sweets, or any other small plastic boxes in which an air-vent can be made.

Various aromatic substances which will be placed in the boxes: e.g. coffee grains, tea, orange peel, bits of apple, and small pieces of soap.

Aromatic liquids (e.g. perfume, after-shave, Dettol) can be dropped on cotton wool and stored in the boxes.

PROCEDURE

Bring each of the boxes to the children's nose. If possible, clasp their hands round a box and bring hands and box to the nose.

If children have begun to explore their surroundings, have the boxes near them, and let them explore them of their own accord.

Talk to the children about the smells. Make some special comment if the children react strongly to any particular smell. Say things like 'You liked that one!' or 'That was nasty!'

TEACHING HINTS

1 Five to ten minutes of this activity will be sufficient at any one time.
2 Put the boxes away in a cupboard when they are not in use, so that they retain some novelty value.

3 Replace substances, such as pieces of apple, before they have gone 'off'.
4 If children who are mobile try to empty a box, secure it with strong sticky tape. If necessary, bore holes in the box to let the smells escape.
5 Note if the child reacts strongly to any smell.

RECORD-KEEPING

Use a diary or day-sheet (p. 281).

MOVING ON

Move on if children join in the activity of their own accord.

Look at some of the easier activities between pp. 77 and 140, for example, the activities on pp. 77, 87, 109, 121, and 131.

Look also at the most simple activities for developing recognition of sounds (pp. 141–54).

LESS DIFFICULT ACTIVITIES

This activity is at the lower end of the range covered by *Early Communicative Skills*. The remainder of the activities in this section are between pages 27 and 76.

See also Jeffree, McConkey, and Hewson (1977a) and Stevens (1976).

Stimulating the sense of taste

AIM

To let children experience a variety of flavours.

SUITABILITY

The activity is suitable for
- the most profoundly handicapped children.
- children with severe visual impairment.
- children at Stage 1 (p. 15) of our scheme for the development of communication.

MATERIALS

Droppers with rubber bulbs (if possible); alternatively, tea-spoons.
Food and drink with bitter tastes: black coffee, Indian tonic water, olives.
Food and drink with sour tastes: vinegar, PLJ.
Food and drink with sweet tastes: ice-cream, lemonade.
Food and drink with salty tastes: crisps, Tuc biscuits.

PROCEDURE

Check with a parent, doctor, or nurse that there are no foods which the children cannot or should not swallow.

If you are working with fluids, squeeze small quantities from a dropper on to the children's tongue. Note if you get a strong reaction, e.g. from Marmite.

Talk to the children, especially if they react strongly. Say things like 'You liked that one!' or 'That was nasty!'

If you are working with solid foods, place very small quantities on their tongue to avoid the risk of choking.

TEACHING HINTS

1 Note any apparent likes, dislikes, and other strong reactions.
2 This activity can last for five to ten minutes at a time.

RECORD-KEEPING

Use a diary to keep note of any interesting reactions.

MOVING ON

Children who make definite reactions to some substances could be introduced to some of the easier activities between pp. 77 and 140; the activities on pages 77, 87, 109, 121, and 131 are possible examples.

Look also at the most simple activities for developing recognition of sounds (pp. 141–54).

LESS DIFFICULT ACTIVITIES

This activity is at the lower end of the range covered by *Early Communicative Skills*. The remainder of the activities in this section are between pages 27 and 74.

See also Jeffree, McConkey, and Hewson (1977a) and Stevens (1976).

Watching and finding things
Peek-a-boo, played by an adult

AIM

To help the children to follow movement.
To help the children realize that things still exist when they have gone out of sight.

SUITABILITY

The activity is suitable for children who
• take an interest in their surroundings.
• are clearly awake and responsive.
• do not understand language yet.
• are at Stage 2 (p. 17) of our scheme for the development of communication.
  The activity is not suitable for children who are
• blind.
• so profoundly handicapped that they seem to be asleep.

MATERIALS

Sheets of cardboard or strong paper approximately 60 cm x 60 cm.
Large towel.

PROCEDURE

Catch the children's gaze. When you have it, move slowly out of their line of vision. If children lie on a cot or mattress for most of the day, you can do this by dropping down below the level at which they are lying.

If they are in a chair you can hide by holding the cardboard in front of your face, or covering your head with a towel or by vanishing into your pullover.

Look at the children's eyes as you disappear.

If they try to follow you part of the way, they have some skill at tracking. Discover how far they can follow you, and try to increase this gradually.

Move more slowly out of sight at the time you would expect them to lose interest. If their eyes do not follow you, move only very slightly out of their direct gaze.

Encourage any hint of an attempt to follow you.

Reappear suddenly, and say 'Peek-a-boo', 'Hello', or something similar.

Five minutes of this activity at any one time should be enough. Some children are happy to play it for much longer, but this may make them tire of it more quickly in the long run.

TEACHING HINTS

1 Encourage any attempt the children make to follow you with their gaze. Praise them, or make funny faces or noises to hold their attention.
2 Encourage any attempts the children make to join in the game (see p. 79).
3 If necessary, make the activity easier by moving only a little out of the centre of the children's gaze, or by moving very slowly.

RECORD-KEEPING

Use a diary or day-sheet (p. 281).

MOVING ON

Move to more difficult activities
• if the children enjoy peek-a-boo.
• if the children's gaze follows your movement easily.
 Tackle any of the other non-verbal activities which are still quite hard; you will find them between pp. 79 and 140.
 Look also at 'Recognizing and understanding sounds' (pp. 141–54) and 'Imitating actions' and 'Imitating vocal sounds' (pp. 155–67).

LESS DIFFICULT ACTIVITIES

If the child shows no interest in this activity, look instead at:
• activities for stimulating their vision (pp. 41–8).
• activities for stimulating their hearing (pp. 27–40).
• activities for stimulating their sense of touch (pp. 49–56).

Watching and finding things
Peek-a-boo, played by the child

AIM

To help the children realize that things still exist when they have gone from sight.

SUITABILITY

The activity is suitable for children who
• take an interest in their surroundings.
• are clearly awake and responsive.
• do not understand language yet.
• are at Stage 2 (p. 17) of our scheme for the development of communication.
  The activity is not suitable for children who are
• very severely visually impaired.
• so profoundly handicapped that they often seem to be asleep.

MATERIALS

A towel, or piece of cloth of similar size to a towel.

PROCEDURE

Wait until the children are in a reasonably contented mood.
  Say 'Bye-bye' (or something similar) and cover their head with the towel.
  Say 'Peek-a-boo', or 'Hello', and pull it off again.
  When the children seem used to the activity, begin helping them to pull off the towel of their own accord.
  If the activity seems to mystify them at the start, do not cover their eyes entirely with the towel. Lift it up in front of them just until you disappear from view, then lower it again. Or drape it on their head, lower an edge down past the eyes, then lift it up again quickly.
  Five minutes of this activity at any one time should be enough.

TEACHING HINTS

1 Do not continue with this activity if the children seem distressed by it.
2 Encourage and assist any attempts they make to remove the towel.
3 When the towel is finally off, show the children that you are pleased.

RECORD-KEEPING

Use a diary or day-sheet (p. 281).

MOVING ON

Move on if the children pull off the towel of their own accord.

Tackle any of the other non-verbal activities which are still quite hard; you will find them between pp. 51 and 140.

Look also at 'Recognizing and understanding sounds' (pp. 141–54) and 'Imitating actions' and 'Imitating vocal sounds' (pp. 155–67).

LESS DIFFICULT ACTIVITIES

If the child shows no interest in this activity, look instead at
- the simpler form of peek-a-boo which appears on p. 77.
- activities for stimulating their vision (pp. 41–8).
- activities for stimulating their hearing (pp. 27–40).
- activities for stimulating their sense of touch (pp. 49–56).

Watching and finding things
Finding half-hidden objects

AIM

The children will realize that things continue to exist even when they have gone out of sight.

SUITABILITY

The activity is suitable for children who
• take an interest in their surroundings.
• do not understand language yet.
• are at Stage 2 (p. 17) of our scheme for the development of communication.
  The activity is not suitable for children who are
• very severely visually impaired.
• so profoundly handicapped that they often seem to be asleep.

MATERIALS

Toys which the children like.
Toys which produce a distinct noise (powered by clockwork or battery).
Screens, shoe-box, opaque plastic containers, cocoa tins, pieces of cloth.

PROCEDURE

(a) Partly cover a Teddy bear with a towel so that its feet, head, and ears remain visible.
    Discover how much of the bear you have to uncover before the children recognize it and pull off the rest of the towel.
    Through play, give them any help you can. For example, let them see you covering the bear and then quickly uncover it again. Or put one of the ends of the towel in their hand, and help them to pull it away.
(b) Remove one end from a shoe-box and turn it upside down to form a garage. How far out of the garage must a car be, before the children take an interest in it?
    Gradually increase the amount by which you conceal it. Eventually they should retrieve it even after it has been completely garaged.
(c) Let the bowl (or handle) of a spoon protrude from some opaque container. How much of the spoon must protrude before the children will pull it out?

TEACHING HINTS

1 Store away the materials for this exercise after you have used them. This may help to keep the children interested in them if they like them in the first place.
2 Make the activities more amusing by making animal or vehicle noises, as appropriate.
3 Toys which will make sounds can be useful. They still clearly exist even when they are covered up completely.

RECORD-KEEPING

Use a diary or day-sheet (p. 281).

MOVING ON

Move to the activity concerned with completely hidden objects (p. 83) when the child has no trouble finding the partly hidden ones.

LESS DIFFICULT ACTIVITIES

If the child shows little interest in objects when they are partly hidden, look at
• activities for stimulating the sense of vision (pp. 41–8).
• early activities in the 'purposeful behaviour' section (e.g. p. 109).

Watching and finding things
Finding completely hidden objects

AIM

Children will realize that objects continue to exist even when they have gone out of sight.
Children will start to explore their surroundings.

SUITABILITY

The activity is suitable for children who
- take an interest in their surroundings.
- do not understand language yet.
- uncover partly hidden toys and other objects (activity on p. 81).
- are at Stage 2 (p. 17) of our scheme for the development of communication.
  The activity is not suitable for children who are
- very severely visually impaired.
- so profoundly handicapped that they often seem to be asleep.

MATERIALS

Shoe-box and lid decorated with shiny or patterned paper.
Toy chest.
Pillow-slip, or similar bag.
A selection of toys and other objects likely to interest the child.
The Down Box (p. 199).
The Goodbye–Hello Box (p. 199).

PROCEDURE

(a) Place six or seven objects (e.g. a mirror, a toy car, a soft toy, a squeezy toy, etc.) in the shoe-box.

Help the children to open it, and bring out a toy. Close the box again. Replace that toy with another one from the box after a few minutes. Encourage children to take an interest by joining in the activity with them.

If you think it will help, new objects can be put into the box every few days.

(b) Bring the children to a toy-chest in which some favourite toy is hidden among the contents. Pretend to search hard before you 'find' it.

Show the children that you are pleased if they discover any object they like especially.

83

(c) Give a pillow-case a narrow neck by sewing a band of elastic around the opening.

    The children can be encouraged to look in the pillow-case if you hold it open with both hands.

    They can also put one hand in, and feel around the objects which are concealed.

(d) The Down Box and Goodbye-Hello Box. Let objects vanish and then reappear at a different point.

    To let the children understand this, use a helper to direct the children's attention first at the point of disappearance, and then at the point of reappearance.

TEACHING HINTS

1 Make the activities more interesting by joining in yourself. For example, in (d) you could say 'Bye-bye' or move as an object vanishes, and 'Hello' as it appears again.
2 Show the children that you are pleased if they begin to play with any of the materials of their own accord.

RECORD-KEEPING

Use a diary or day-sheet (p. 281).

MOVING ON

If a child has no difficulty with this activity
- look first at any of the other non-verbal activities which are still quite hard; you will find them between pp. 85 and 140.
- then move to 'Recognizing and understanding sounds' (pp. 141–54) and 'Imitating actions' and 'Imitating vocal sounds' (pp. 155–67).

LESS DIFFICULT ACTIVITIES

If a child continually loses interest in objects when they have disappeared from view, try some activities in which the disappearance is not complete, e.g. p. 81.

Watching and finding things
Objects that disappear

AIM

To help children understand that an object still exists after it has gone out of sight.
To encourage children to follow a moving object with their gaze.
To encourage children to guess where a vanishing object may reappear.

SUITABILITY

Children are ready for this activity if they
- take an interest in their surroundings.
- definitely look at objects occasionally.
- show excitement or pleasure when you go to work with them.
- try to reach out for objects.
- do not understand language yet.
- are in the early part of Stage 2 (p. 17) of our scheme for the development of communication.
  It is not suitable for children who are
- very severely visually impaired.
- so profoundly handicapped that they often appear to be asleep.

MATERIALS

Cars and other wheeled toys attached to strings.
A screen — a large book or a cardboard box will do.

PROCEDURE

Choose a wheeled toy which you think the children will like. Catch their attention. If necessary, turn them physically to look at what you are doing. Tow the toy across the line of vision. Encourage them to keep looking at it by making appropriate animal or vehicle noises. Show them that you are pleased if they do look at it.

When the children follow the moving toy with their eyes, add the following complication: put the screen between yourself and the children; let them see the toy, then tow it out of sight behind the screen.

If children lose interest when the toy goes out of sight, turn their gaze to where it will reappear. The help of another adult is useful for this.

TEACHING HINTS

1 Try the following tactics if you do not succeed at first:
   • bring the toy and screen nearer to the children;
   • make the screen smaller so that part of the toy is always exposed;
   • use a shorter screen (or pull the toy more quickly) so that the toy does not vanish for so long;
   • use a larger toy;
   • let the children see behind the screen;
   • say 'Here it comes!' just before the toy reappears.
2 Give less help as the children begin to get the idea.

RECORD-KEEPING

Keep notes on a day-sheet (p. 281).

MOVING ON

Move on
• if the children move their gaze from the vanishing point to the reappearance point without any help.
• if the children push the screen aside to get at the vanished toy.
   First make sure that they can carry out most of the harder pre-verbal activities between pp. 87 and 140. Then look at 'Recognizing and understanding sounds' (pp. 141–54) and 'Imitating actions' and 'Imitating vocal sounds' (pp. 155–67).

LESS DIFFICULT ACTIVITIES

If the children lose interest in the toy when it vanishes
• remain at the earlier stage of this activity — concentrate on catching and holding their attention with toys, other objects, and activities which seem to interest them.
• try the simpler version of peek-a-boo (p. 77).

Handling objects
Patting with the hand

AIM

Children will hit or pat objects with their hands.

SUITABILITY

The activity is suitable for children who
• hold objects in their hands quite firmly.
• hold objects and look at them.
• are at Stage 2 (p. 17) of our scheme for the development of communication.
  The activity is not suitable for children who
• are so profoundly handicapped that they often seem to be asleep.
• are advanced enough to be able to handle objects in more complicated ways,
  such as crumpling, stretching, or swinging.

MATERIALS

Soft toys, rag-dolls, sponges, hairbrushes, or any other soft object that the child
can hold.
    Lightweight percussion instruments, baking-trays, stiff cardboard boxes, or
any other objects that make an interesting sound when struck by hand.

PROCEDURE

Choose objects that you think the children will like.
    Play with the objects, bringing them gently to touch the children if they are
soft, or striking them to make a sound if they are resonant.
    Encourage any attempt the children make to play with the object of their own
accord.
    If necessary, give them some help to produce an action of patting or striking.
    Talk about what you are doing to hold their interest.
    Five to ten minutes of this activity should be possible at any one time.

TEACHING HINTS

1 This activity is well below the level at which exact imitation can be expected.
  Do not worry if a child does not produce good copies of your actions.
2 Don't clutter the work area with too many different toys.

87

3 If children develop a special liking for some toys in the course of the activity, help to keep them special by storing them away when you have finished.
4 Sit, holding the children, if this closer contact gives you better results.

RECORD-KEEPING

Use a diary or day-sheet (p. 281).

MOVING ON

Move on when children spontaneously hit or pat objects with their hands.
  Look at
- similar activities on pp. 89–92.
- slightly more complicated activities on pp. 93-108.
- other non-verbal activities (from pp. 109–40).
- recognition of sounds (pp. 141–54).

LESS DIFFICULT ACTIVITIES

If the children do not hit or pat objects with their hands, look at activities for stimulating the sense of touch (pp. 49–56) and watch out for any responses the children make in them.

Handling objects
Percussion toys for shaking

AIM

Children will shake small objects that they can lift up.

SUITABILITY

The activity is suitable for children who
● hold objects in their hands.
● hold objects and look at them.
● are at Stage 2 (p. 17) of our scheme for the development of communication.
The activity is not suitable for children who
● are so profoundly handicapped that they often seem to be asleep.
● handle objects in more complicated ways, such as crumpling, stretching, or swinging.

MATERIALS

Rattles.
Small tambourines.
Tins and polythene containers holding peas, rice, or barley.
Bells.

PROCEDURE

Work with objects which you think the children will like. Play with the objects, letting the children hear the range of sounds that can be produced.

Talk to them, and make gestures, to make the activity more interesting.

Encourage any attempt they make to pick up or shake the objects of their own accord.

If necessary, put the object in their hands and help them to go through the action of shaking.

Five to ten minutes at a time can be spent on this activity.

TEACHING HINTS

1 Do not try to force the children into shaking the objects. They are more likely to succeed if they make the first move, even if you have to help them along afterwards.

2 This activity is well below the level at which exact imitation can be expected. Do not worry if the children do not produce good copies of your actions.
3 If the children develop a special liking for some toy in the course of the activity, help to keep it special by storing it away when you have finished.
4 Sit, holding the children from behind, if this closer contact brings better results.

RECORD-KEEPING

Use a diary or day-sheet (p. 281).

MOVING ON

Move on when the children shake objects of their own accord.
   Look at
- similar activities on pp. 87–92.
- slightly more complicated activities on pp. 93–108.
- other non-verbal activities (from pp. 109–40).
- recognition of sounds (pp. 141–54).

LESS DIFFICULT ACTIVITIES

If a child does not begin to shake objects, look at
- patting with the hand (p. 87).
- early activities in the 'purposeful behaviour' section (e.g. p. 109).

Handling objects
Dangling toys

AIM

The children will hit objects hanging from the ceiling to make them swing to and fro.

SUITABILITY

The activity is suitable for children who
- pick up objects and look at them closely.
- deliberately knock two objects together.
- are at Stage 2 (p. 17) of our scheme for the development of communication.
  The activity is not suitable for children who
- do not pick up objects.
- play at more advanced levels, such as make-believe.

MATERIALS

Woollen pom-poms, dolls, bags, or plastic containers filled with dried peas. String or elastic to suspend these objects from the ceiling.

PROCEDURE

The children may play with these materials spontaneously.

If not, push one towards them when they are a few steps away from you, and see what happens.

Praise any attempts they make to join in. Later on, this can become a game played between two people.

If necessary, help them to make the necessary pushing or hitting movements.

TEACHING HINTS

1 If possible, do not leave hanging toys on display all the time. They are likely to lose their power of attraction, and they may distract attention from other teaching materials.
2 Some children spin hanging toys as a sort of ritualistic behaviour. You can discourage this by putting the toys away when not in use and by encouraging the children's attempts to make the objects swing instead of spin.

RECORD-KEEPING

Diary or day-sheet.

MOVING ON

Move on when a child makes the hanging toys swing by hitting or pushing them.
  Look at
- make-believe play (pp. 168–75).
- recognition of sounds (pp. 141–54).
- imitation (pp. 155–67).

LESS DIFFICULT ACTIVITIES

If this activity is too difficult for a child, look instead at the early activities in the
sections on 'purposeful behaviour' (p. 109) and 'making things happen' (p. 121).

Handling objects
Objects that slide about

AIM

The children will make objects slide about on a surface.

SUITABILITY

The activity is suitable for children who
• pick up objects and look at them closely.
• deliberately knock two objects together.
• are at Stage 2 (p. 17) of our scheme for the development of communication.
  The activity is not suitable for children who
• do not pick up objects.
• have moved on to more advanced levels of play, such as make-believe.

MATERIALS

Surfaces: floor, table, sand-tray, corrugated polythene sheeting.
Objects: towels, paper, sponge-rubber, books, egg-boxes.

PROCEDURE

Catch the children's attention and slide a piece of cloth, for example, along the floor or table as if it were a model car.
  Encourage the children to join in, and praise any attempts that they make.
  Use a variety of surfaces and objects, so that the children find that some objects are easy to slide while others are difficult.
  Five to ten minutes at a time can be spent on this activity.

TEACHING HINTS

Make vehicle noises, or any other sounds that may appeal to the children.

RECORD-KEEPING

Use a diary or day-sheet (p. 281).

MOVING ON

If a child does slide objects around on surfaces, look at
- make-believe play (pp. 168–75).
- recognition of sounds (pp. 141–54).
- imitation (pp. 155–67).

LESS DIFFICULT ACTIVITIES

If the child has difficulty with this activity, look at the early activities in the sections on 'purposeful behaviour' (p. 109) and 'making things happen' (p. 121).

Handling objects
Examining objects closely

AIM

The children will make a close examination of objects using hands, eyes, and nose.

SUITABILITY

The activity is suitable for children who
• pick up objects.
• knock objects together.
• hit objects against a surface.
• are at Stage 2 (p. 17) of our scheme for the development of communication.
  The activity is not suitable for children who
• do not reach out for objects.
• have moved on to more advanced levels of play, such as make-believe.

MATERIALS

Objects with interesting textures: sponges, hairbrushes, sandpaper, balloons.
Objects with interesting smells: flowers, perfume bottles.
Objects with interesting shapes and/or colours: containers for school pens, scissors-boxes, egg whisks, potato-mashers, safety mirrors.
Objects which stimulate several senses: musical boxes, Kelly toys (which bob back when knocked over).

PROCEDURE

Give the children a variety of objects (one at a time) which you think will interest them.

They may inspect an object on their own by looking at it, turning it over, pulling at it, prodding it, sniffing it, and so on. Encourage them if you see this.

If they do not play with it of their own accord, bring the object to them and explore it together. Draw their attention to any interesting aspects such as smell or texture.

Talk about the activity to make it more interesting.

Five to ten minutes at a time can be spent on this activity.

TEACHING HINTS

1 Change the objects for inspection fairly regularly.
2 The activity need not be part of your teaching plan if children inspect things of their own accord.

RECORD-KEEPING

Use a diary or day-sheet (p. 281).

MOVING ON

Move on if a child does inspect objects closely.
   Look at
● more advanced activities in handling (pp. 97–108).
● recognition of sounds (pp. 141–54).

LESS DIFFICULT ACTIVITIES

If children do not inspect objects closely even after you have given them a lot of encouragement, look at pp. 87–94, and at the early activities in the sections on 'purposeful behaviour' (p. 109) and 'making things happen' (p. 121).

Handling objects
Using objects as hammers and drumsticks

AIM

The children will hit objects against a surface.

SUITABILITY

The activity is suitable for children who
- hold objects in their hands.
- hold objects and look at them.
- are at Stage 2 (p. 17) of our scheme for the development of communication.
  The activity is not suitable for children who
- are so profoundly handicapped that they often seem to be asleep.
- handle objects in more complicated ways, such as crumpling, stretching, or swinging.

MATERIALS

Surfaces polythene-covered mattresses, table-tops, base of the sand-tray, tea-trays, sheets of brown paper.
Beaters cutlery, drumsticks, plastic hammers, dolls, anything else that the child can hold.

PROCEDURE

Work with beaters and surfaces which you think the children will like.

Catch the children's attention and play with the beater yourself. Increase interest in the activity by talking about it and by your gestures.

Give the children a beater of their own, and encourage any attempt they make to use it.

If necessary, give them some help to make the action of beating.

Five minutes of this activity at any one time should be sufficient.

TEACHING HINTS

1 This activity is well below the level at which exact imitation can be expected. Do not worry if the children do not produce good copies of your actions.
2 If the children develop a special liking for some toy in the course of the activity, help to keep it special by storing it away when you have finished.

3 Sit, holding the children from behind, if this closer contact gives you better results.

RECORD-KEEPING

Use a diary or day-sheet (p. 281).

MOVING ON

Move on when children hit objects against surfaces of their own accord.
   Look at
- similar activities on pp. 99–102.
- slightly more complicated activities on pp. 103–8.
- other non-verbal activities (e.g. pp. 85, 117, 131).
- recognition of sounds (pp. 141–54).

LESS DIFFICULT ACTIVITIES

If a child does not begin to hit objects against a surface, look at
- more simple ways of manipulating objects (pp. 87–94).
- early activities in the section on 'purposeful behaviour' (p. 109).

Handling objects
Toys that can be waved or shaken

AIM

The children will wave objects in the air.

SUITABILITY

The activity is suitable for children who
- hold objects in their hands.
- hold objects and look at them.
- are at Stage 2 (p. 17) of our scheme for the development of communication.
  The activity is not suitable for children who
- are so profoundly handicapped that they often seem to be asleep.
- handle objects in more complicated ways, such as crumpling, stretching, or
  swinging.

MATERIALS

Sticks with ribbons or streamers attached.
'Snow' scenes in water-filled containers.
Rattles enclosing spinning discs.

PROCEDURE

Work with toys which you think the children will like. Play with the toys, drawing attention to any attractive movement. Increase your chances of keeping them
interested by talking about what is going on and by gesture.

Encourage the children to join in, by giving them a toy of their own or the
one you have been holding.

If necessary, put it in their hand and help them to wave it in their field of vision.
Five to ten minutes at a time can be spent on this activity. *244607*

TEACHING HINTS

1 Do not force children into waving. They are more likely to succeed if they
   make the first move, even if you have to help them along afterwards.
2 This activity is well below the level at which exact imitation can be expected.
   Aim to get the children into action, rather than to copy your actions precisely.
3 If the children develop a liking for some toy in the course of the activity, help

to keep it special by storing it away when you have finished.
4 Sit, holding the children from behind, if this closer contact brings better results.

RECORD-KEEPING

Use a diary or day-sheet (p. 281).

MOVING ON

Move on when children wave objects of their own accord.
Look at
- similar activities on pp. 101–2.
- slightly more complicated activities on pp. 103–8.
- other non-verbal activities (e.g. pp. 85, 117, 131).
- recognition of sounds (pp. 141–54).

LESS DIFFICULT ACTIVITIES

If children do not wave objects of their own accord, look at
- more simple ways of manipulating objects (pp. 87–94).
- early activities in the section on purposeful behaviour (p. 109).

Handling objects
Objects that can be squeezed

AIM

The child will manipulate flexible objects in a variety of ways, such as crumpling.

SUITABILITY

The activity is suitable for children who
• pick up objects and look at them closely.
• deliberately knock two objects together.
• are at Stage 2 (p. 17) of our scheme for the development of communication.
  The activity is not suitable for children who
• do not pick up objects.
• have moved on to more advanced levels of play, such as make-believe.

MATERIALS

Blank newsprint, crinkly paper from biscuit boxes, baking foil, pieces of cloth, sponges.
Paper balloons (see Van Witsen 1967: 71, for directions on how to make an origami balloon).

PROCEDURE

Play with the materials and encourage the children to join in by drawing attention to the change in shape and to any other interesting effects. For example,
• biscuit-box paper and foil will produce a good sound when crumpled.
• a sponge will shed water when it is squeezed.
  Ten minutes at a time could be spent on this activity.

TEACHING HINTS

1 Stop the activity before the children tire of it.
2 Store away the materials when they are not in use to keep them special.

RECORD-KEEPING

Use a diary or day-sheet (p. 281).

MOVING ON

Move on when a child crumples paper and similar materials easily. Look at
- make-believe play (pp. 168–75).
- recognition of sounds (pp. 141–54).
- imitation (pp. 155–67).

LESS DIFFICULT ACTIVITIES

If the child does not begin to join in this activity, look at the early activities in the
sections on 'purposeful behaviour' (p. 109) and 'making things happen' (p. 121).

Handling objects
Hitting two objects together

AIM

The children will hit two objects together.

SUITABILITY

The activity is suitable for children who
- hold objects in their hands.
- hold objects and look at them.
- occasionally hit objects against a surface.
- are at Stage 2 (p. 17) of our scheme for the development of communication.
  The activity is not suitable for children who
- are so profoundly handicapped that they often seem to be asleep.
- handle objects in more complicated ways, such as crumpling, stretching, or
  swinging.

MATERIALS

Beaters and drums (or tambourines, biscuit-tins, polythene containers, cardboard
  boxes, etc.).
Pieces of wood for striking against each other.
Small metal trays, or any other kind of containers which can be held easily and
  struck against each other.

PROCEDURE

Work with objects which you think the children will like.

Hold the objects, one in each hand, and strike them against each other, making
sure that the children can see you. Encourage any attempt they make to join in.

If necessary, put an object in each of their hands and help them to strike them
together. Praise any effort which seems to be getting nearer the complete action.

Five minutes of this activity may be sufficient at any one time.

TEACHING HINTS

1 This activity is well below the level at which exact imitation can be expected.
  Do not worry if the children do not produce good copies of your action.
2 If children develop a special liking for some toy in the course of the activity,

help to keep it special by storing it away when you have finished.
3 Sit, holding the children from behind, if this closer contact brings better results.

RECORD-KEEPING

Use a diary or day-sheet (p. 281).

MOVING ON

Move on when children are able to strike the objects together of their own accord.
Look at
• similar activities on pp. 105–8.
• other non-verbal activities (pp. 85, 117, 131).
• recognition of sounds (pp. 141–54).

LESS DIFFICULT ACTIVITIES

If a child does not begin to play with the two objects together, look at more simple
ways of manipulating objects (pp. 85–102).

Handling objects
Materials for stretching and tearing

AIM

The children will learn that some objects can be stretched out and that a few of them can be torn.

SUITABILITY

The activity is suitable for children who
• pick up objects and look at them closely.
• deliberately knock two objects together.
• are at Stage 2 (p. 17) of our scheme for the development of communication.
  The activity is not suitable for children who
• do not pick up objects.
• have moved on to more advanced levels of play, such as make-believe.

MATERIALS

Newspaper, pieces of cloth, woollen clothing, or other clothing which is springy.

PROCEDURE

You could introduce tearing and stretching by placing one end of the material in the children's hand and the other in your own. Pull to stretch or rip the material. Increase the children's interest by showing surprise and by talking about what is happening.
   Encourage any attempts they make to pull and tear of their own accord.

TEACHING HINTS

1 Do not leave important papers lying around.
2 The children may not be able to take part in the tug-of-war which is suggested above. In that case, show them what can be done, or take their hands and guide them through the action.

RECORD-KEEPING

Use a diary or day-sheet (p. 281).

MOVING ON

Move on when children stretch or tear things of their own accord. Discourage tearing by finding more interesting activities to take its place.

Look at
- make-believe play (pp. 168–75).
- recognition of sounds (pp. 141–54)
- imitation (pp. 155–67)

LESS DIFFICULT ACTIVITIES

If the children do not begin to take an interest in pulling and stretching materials, look at the early activities in the sections on 'purposeful behaviour' (p. 109) and 'making things happen' (p. 121).

Handling objects
Filling and emptying containers

AIM

The children will fill containers with a variety of substances.

SUITABILITY

The activity is suitable for children who
- pick up objects and look at them closely.
- deliberately knock two objects together.
- are at Stage 2 (p. 17) of our scheme for the development of communication.
  The activity is not suitable for children who
- do not pick up objects.
- have moved on to more advanced levels of play, such as make-believe.

MATERIALS

Containers: cups, bowls, jugs, boxes.
Substances for placing in containers: sand, water, buttons, bricks, Unifix, small
   toys, beads.

PROCEDURE

Work with materials which you think will interest the children.

Show them that substances can be dropped or poured into a variety of containers.

Encourage them to take part, help them if necessary, and praise any attempts that they make.

Ten minutes can be spent on this activity at any one time.

TEACHING HINTS

You may decide to use a spoon to transfer substances into the containers. Do not be surprised if the children cannot do this.

RECORD-KEEPING

Use a diary or day-sheet (p. 281).

MOVING ON

Move on when the child places substances inside containers during free play.
  Look at
- make-believe play (pp. 168–75).
- recognition of sounds (pp. 141–54).
- imitation (pp. 155–67)

LESS DIFFICULT ACTIVITIES

If the child does not begin to take an interest in filling and emptying containers, look at more simple ways of handling objects (pp. 87–106).

Behaving purposefully
Objects that can be held in the hand

AIM

To encourage the children to hold interesting objects.

SUITABILITY

The activity is suitable for children who
- take an interest in their surroundings.
- are clearly awake and responsive.
- do not understand language yet.
- are in the early part of Stage 2 (p. 17) of our scheme for the development of communication.
    The activity is not suitable for children who are so profoundly handicapped that they seem to be asleep.

MATERIALS

Hand-shaken musical toys.
Light percussion instruments.
Mirror.
Dolls, cars, or any other favourite toys.

PROCEDURE

Show one of the toys to the children in as many ways as possible:
- let them hear any sounds it makes.
- let them see its movement, bright colours, striking pattern, or prominent parts.
- let them feel the toy.
    Encourage any movement which suggests that a child is trying to hold the toy deliberately.
    This activity can last for five to ten minutes at a time.

TEACHING HINTS

1 The aim of this activity is very simple indeed — you just want the children to hold the toy. Reaching out for it is more difficult, and appears later in the book (p. 111).

2 Guide the children's hands on to the toy if necessary. Gradually fade out this help until they themselves close their fingers over it.
3 Make allowances, of course, for physically handicapped children who do not have a good hand-grip.

RECORD-KEEPING

Use a diary or day-sheeet (p. 281).

MOVING ON

Move on to activities on reaching (pp. 111, 113, 115) when the child holds things in a deliberate way.

LESS DIFFICULT ACTIVITIES

If a child does not begin to grasp objects with any sense of purpose, look at
• activities for stimulating the sense of touch (pp. 49–56).
• activities for stimulating vision (pp. 41–8).
• activities for stimulating hearing (pp. 27–40).

Behaving purposefully
Reaching for objects

AIM

Children will reach out to grasp objects that they want.

SUITABILITY

The activity is suitable for children who
- take an interest in their surroundings.
- hold or pick up objects.
- do not understand language yet.
- are at Stage 2 (p. 17) of our scheme for the development of communication.
  The activity is not suitable for
- some children who are severely physically handicapped.
- children who are so profoundly handicapped that they often seem to be asleep.

MATERIALS

Hand-shaken musical toys.
Lightweight percussion instruments.
Mirror.
Dolls, cars, or any other favourite toys.

PROCEDURE

Play with the children, using a toy you want them to reach for. Make it 'walk' or roll along near them, and make any sound effects (such as animal and vehicle noises) which you think will catch their interest.

After a little, place it at the limit of their reach along the floor or table.

If they make a complaining sound, that is good as they are communicating! However, encourage them to reach for the toy, helping them if necessary by bringing it nearer or by bringing their arm out to it.

When they get the idea of the activity, gradually place it beyond reach so that they have to try harder before they can grasp it.

TEACHING HINTS

1 Encourage any efforts a child makes to reach out for the object.

2 It may help to keep some objects especially for this activity and to store them away afterwards.

RECORD-KEEPING

Use a diary or day-sheet (p. 281).

MOVING ON

Move on to some of the harder pre-verbal activities between pp. 77 and 140 when children reach (of their own accord) for things that they want.

LESS DIFFICULT ACTIVITIES

If a child does not begin to reach out for objects, look at
- activities for stimulating vision (pp. 41–8).
- activities for stimulating hearing (pp. 27–40).
- activities for stimulating sense of touch (pp. 49–56).
- activities for stimulating sense of movement (pp. 57–66).

Behaving purposefully
Reaching out to be lifted

AIM

Children will hold out their arms to be lifted.

SUITABILITY

The activity is suitable for children who
- are clearly awake and responsive.
- do not understand language yet.
- are at Stage 2 (p. 17) of our scheme for the development of communication.

The activity is not suitable for children who are so profoundly handicapped that they often seem to be asleep.

The activity will have to be adapted for children who are so severely physically handicapped that they cannot hold out their arms.

MATERIALS

None.

PROCEDURE

Do not attempt to lift children if you are likely to injure them or yourself.

Approach the children as if you are going to pick them up. This will probably happen several times in the course of a normal day.

Wait to see if they make any movement which suggests that they know they are going to be lifted. If they do, show them that you are pleased and lift them up directly.

Next time, wait until their movement is slightly more obvious before you act. Very gradually, draw the children out to the kind of action you want from them. Physically able children should be able to stretch out their arms, but children with cerebral palsy may be capable of much less movement.

Read Nancy Finnie's (1974) book for advice on handling children with cerebral palsy.

TEACHING HINTS

1 Treat any sounds the children make during this activity *as if* they are attempts

to make you act. Later you may be able to shape them into words. (For a more advanced use of *as if* behaviour see p. 191).

2 Show the children that you are pleased if they pull at your clothing rather than reach out. This is quite an advanced form of communication.

RECORD-KEEPING

Use a diary. Note the date when you begin this activity. Note any significant changes afterwards.

MOVING ON

If children do hold out their hands to be lifted, try some of the more difficult pre-verbal activities between pp. 77 and 140. Also, look at 'Imitating actions' and 'Imitating vocal sounds' (pp. 155–67), and 'Recognizing and understanding sounds' (pp. 141–54).

LESS DIFFICULT ACTIVITIES

If children do not hold out their arms to be lifted, try a more simple activity for helping to reach for things (pp. 109–12).

Behaving purposefully
Reaching for food

AIM

The children will reach out to obtain food and drink.

SUITABILITY

The activity is suitable for children who
- can take a hold of objects.
- pick up toys near them.
- do not understand language yet.
- are at Stage 2 (p. 17) of our scheme for the development of communication.
    The activity is not suitable for children who are so profoundly handicapped that they often seem to be asleep.

MATERIALS

Pieces of solid food, e.g. bananas or cake.
Softer food (in a bowl), eaten with spoon.
Drink in a cup.

PROCEDURE

Make sure that it is safe to feed the children the food you intend to use.

Carry out this activity at some appropriate time such as the mid-morning break. Place the food just within the children's reach. If using soft food in a bowl, put the spoon in their hand.
    Encourage any movement which suggests that they are trying to reach for the food. Praise their efforts, and help them if necessary by bringing the food nearer to their hand. Help them to hold spoons or drinking mugs.
    Gradually fade out assistance until the children do all the reaching of their own accord.

TEACHING HINTS

This is not an exercise in learning to feed. Help the children in any way on the 'return journey' from food to mouth.
    For advice on feeding, see Anderson (1983), Kiernan, Jordan, and Saunders (1978), and Warner (1981).

RECORD-KEEPING

Use a diary or day-sheet (p. 281).

MOVING ON

There is no point in continuing with this exercise after the children have managed it successfully a few times.

Discover if they will make vocal sounds in addition (or instead of) pointing (p. 119).

LESS DIFFICULT ACTIVITIES

If the child does not attempt to reach out for food, make sure that they have had experience of picking up objects and handling them (pp. 109–12).

Behaving purposefully
Toys on strings

AIM

Children will use strings attached to toys to bring them to them.

SUITABILITY

The activity is suitable for children who
• reach out for objects.
• do not understand language yet.
• are at Stage 2 (p. 17) of our scheme for the development of communication.
    The activity is not suitable for children who are not grasping objects of their own accord.

MATERIALS

Any small toys which can be pulled along on a string.

PROCEDURE

Make sure the children have seen you pulling along and reeling in objects tied to a string.
    Sit with the children. Place the string in their hand and help them to reel in the string.
    Encourage any movement they make which brings the object nearer to them. Give less assistance as the children's performance improves.

TEACHING HINTS

1 The string will be one of the first tools the children have come across. Shorten it if they do not get the idea.
2 Change the toy for a possibly more attractive one if they show little interest in the activity. A brighter toy, a favourite one, or one which makes a sound may help.
3 Change the thickness of string if the original one is difficult to grasp.
4 Talk to the children about what is going on. Phrases like 'Here it comes!', 'Pull! Pull!', or 'See the car!' would be suitable.

RECORD-KEEPING

Use a day-sheet (p. 281).

MOVING ON

Move on when the children clearly understand that they can use the string to pull objects towards them.

Look at some of the harder non-verbal activities between pp. 117 and 140.

Look also at 'Recognizing and understanding sounds' (pp. 141-54) and 'Imitating actions' and 'Imitating vocal sounds' (pp. 155-67).

LESS DIFFICULT ACTIVITIES

The children may have trouble realizing that they can use string to pull objects towards them. If so, try the rather easier activities which appear on pp. 109-12.

Behaving purposefully
Pointing or calling out for a purpose

AIM

Children will point or produce sounds to indicate that they want something.

SUITABILITY

The activity is suitable for children who
- take a hold of objects.
- pick up objects near them.
- reach out to pick up things they want.
- do not understand language yet.
- are at Stage 2 (p. 17) of our scheme for the development of communication.

The activity will also be suitable for some alert, but severely physically handicapped children who are unable to grasp or pick up.

The activity is not suitable for children who are so profoundly handicapped that they often seem to be asleep.

MATERIALS

Attractive toys.
Food or drink.

PROCEDURE

The activity is a development of the basic reaching activity (p. 111) and the reaching-for-food exercise (p. 115).

Place the toy or food just outside the children's reach. If they stretch out their arm to its full extent, give the object to them.

If they are very severely physically handicapped, decide on some other movement than 'arm to full extent'. A steady gaze in the right direction may be suitable.

Gradually move the object further away from the children so that they have no chance of being able to stretch to it. Immediately reward any reaching toward the object by bringing it to them.

Give special encouragement to any sound the children make when pointing to the object (or looking at it, in the case of children who are severely physically handicapped).

Once you know that they will make a sound, wait until you hear one on future occasions. Later on you may be able to shape this into a word (p. 206).

TEACHING HINTS

1 Don't set too high standards too soon. Progress very slowly or you may discourage the children.
2 If the children point quite successfully with the whole arm, mould their hand into the normal adult fore-finger point. Make sure that they see you pointing to things also. They may copy you eventually.

RECORD-KEEPING

Use a diary or day-sheet (p. 281).

MOVING ON

Move on when you are confident that the children are pointing in the direction of things that they want, or are making sounds to indicate that they want something.

Try some of the harder pre-verbal activities between pp. 77 and 140. Also, look at 'Imitating actions' and 'Imitating vocal sounds' (pp. 155–67) and 'Recognizing and understanding sounds' (pp. 141–54).

LESS DIFFICULT ACTIVITIES

If this activity is too difficult for the children, make sure that
• they can reach out towards things that they want (p. 111).
• they have had experience of picking up objects and handling them (pp. 87–104).

Making things happen
Knocking down towers of bricks

AIM

Children will knock down towers of bricks of their own accord.

SUITABILITY

The activity is suitable for children who
● are responsive, and interested in the world.
● do not understand language yet.
● are at Stage 2 (p. 17) of our scheme for the development of communication.
    The activity is not suitable for children who are so profoundly handicapped that they often seem to be asleep.

MATERIALS

Building bricks.
Stacking-cups.
Any similar materials which can be built into an unstable tower.

PROCEDURE

Play with the children to show them how the bricks can be built into a tower.
    When it is five or six bricks high, push it over. Make sure you have the children's attention. Make the event as interesting as possible by talking about it (e.g. 'Here it comes!').
    Encourage any attempt the children make to join in the activity. If necessary, guide them through the action of knocking down the tower in the early stages.
    Children will play at this activity for a long time. However, five minutes of it at a time may be enough if you want to sustain their interest.

TEACHING HINTS

1 Let the bricks fall on a padded surface (or stop the activity) if the children show distress.
2 Let the bricks fall on a metal tray if the children do not show much interest.

RECORD-KEEPING

Use a day-sheet (p. 281).

MOVING ON

Move on when the children knock down the tower of their own accord.
Move to other cause-and-effect exercises (pp. 123–31).
Look also at other pre-verbal sections (e.g. between pp. 77 and 140).

LESS DIFFICULT ACTIVITIES

If the children do not knock down towers of bricks of their own accord, look at
• activities for developing reaching (pp. 109–12).
• activities for developing the ability to manipulate objects (pp. 77–92).

Making things happen
Producing interesting sights and sounds

AIM

The children will produce interesting sights and sounds deliberately.

SUITABILITY

The activity is suitable for children who
- reach out for objects.
- do not understand language yet.
- are at Stage 2 (p. 17) of our scheme for the development of communication.

The activity is not suitable for children who are so profoundly handicapped that they often seem to be asleep.

MATERIALS

Toys which make interesting sounds: rattles, bells, drums, plastic or tin containers holding peas, rice, or barley.

Toys which are interesting to look at when struck: streamers on sticks, Fisher Price Activity Centre, coloured balls.

Water-tray, sand-tray.

PROCEDURE

Play with the children to show them the interesting events which can be made to happen when the materials are acted upon. Here are some examples:

Type of action	*Events caused by it*
Patting	Tambourine will sound.
Shaking	Rag-doll's hair will move about, rattle will sound.
Exploring by hand	Balloon will squeak.
Hitting	Water will splash.
	Sand will move about.
	Ball will roll.
Heel-kicking (when lying on back)	Newspaper placed under the feet will crackle.

Encourage any attempt the children make to play with the toys.
If necessary, give them some help to carry out the actions more easily.
Up to ten minutes of this activity can be undertaken at any one time.

TEACHING HINTS

1 This activity is a natural extension of some of the exercises recommended for profoundly handicapped children. However, your aim now is to let the children discover that there are reasons for interesting events taking place.
2 Talk to the children about what is going on, to keep the activity interesting.
3 The equipment may remain interesting for a longer time if it is packed away when not in use.

RECORD-KEEPING

Use a day-sheet (p. 281).

MOVING ON

Move on when
• children pick up toys and play with them of their own accord.
• the children lose interest in the activity.
Look at pp. 121 and 131 for other cause-and-effect exercises.
Look at the harder activities of other pre-verbal sections between pp. 77 and 140.

LESS DIFFICULT ACTIVITIES

If the children do not begin to play with toys (and other objects) of their own accord, look at
• activities for developing reaching (pp. 109–12).
• activities for developing the child's ability to manipulate objects (pp. 77–92).

Making things happen
Simple percussion instruments

AIM

The children will produce interesting sights and sounds deliberately.

SUITABILITY

The activity is suitable for children who
- reach out for objects.
- do not understand language yet.
- are at Stage 2 (p. 17) of our scheme for the development of communication.
  The activity is not suitable for children who are so profoundly handicapped that they often appear to be asleep.

MATERIALS

Small toys suspended on strings. Bright attractive toys and the following sound-producing ones are suitable: commercially produced rattles and bells, home-made items such as plastic or tin containers, holding peas, rice, or barley.
  Crossbar or suspended net to which the strings are attached.

PROCEDURE

Play with the children showing them how the toys can be made to move or sound by striking them.
  Encourage any attempt they make to play with the toys.
  If necessary, give them some help by guiding their arm through the motions of reaching and striking.
  Try attaching an elastic cord from the children's wrist or ankle to the toy to make it move or sound more easily.
  Five to ten minutes of this activity will be sufficient at any one time.

TEACHING HINTS

1 This activity is a natural extension of 'Dangling toys' (p. 91). However, your aim is now to let the children discover that there are reasons for interesting events taking place.
2 Talk to the children about what is going on, to keep the activity interesting.

3 The toys may remain interesting for a longer time if they are packed away
   when not in use.

RECORD-KEEPING

Use a day-sheet (p. 281).

MOVING ON

Move on if
- children hit out at the dangling toys of their own accord.
- children lose interest in the activity.
- children continually prefer to handle or chew the toys rather than strike them.
  Look at pp. 127–30.

LESS DIFFICULT ACTIVITIES

The children may not hit out at the toys even if you help them and even if you
have done your best to make the toys attractive.

   Try the simpler version of this activity which appears on p. 91.

Making things happen
Large toys on wheels

AIM

Children will understand that the toys will move if they kick them along.
Children will understand that their sounds or gestures will make an adult move
   the toys for them.

SUITABILITY

The activity is suitable for children who
• are responsive, and interested in the world.
• do not understand language yet.
• are at Stage 2 (p. 17) of our scheme for the development of communication.
   The activity is not suitable for children who are so profoundly handicapped
that they often seem to be asleep.

MATERIALS

Tyre-on-wheels, large trucks and trains on which the child can sit, go-carts. Details
of commercially made equipment appear in the catalogues of makers of educational equipment (e.g. E.J. Arnold, ESA, Galt).

PROCEDURE

Take the children for a ride on one of the toys.
   Make the activity interesting by talking about what is happening, and varying
the speed and direction of movement.
   Stop after a few seconds, when the children are clearly enjoying the activity.
   Restart if they make some noise or gesture which seems to be 'telling' you
to begin again.
   Encourage any attempts the children make to restart the toy.
   Five to ten minutes at a time are enough to spend on this activity.

TEACHING HINTS

1 Pull the toy along from the front if you think the children do not understand
   that you are pushing it from the back.
2 Children with profound difficulties sometimes enjoy this kind of activity. It
   is really just stimulation of the sense of movement for them, but look out for

any unexpected sounds or movements they may make when you stop.

RECORD-KEEPING

Keep notes in a diary or on a day-sheet (p. 281).

MOVING ON

Move on when
- children are able to make the toys (and themselves) move by kicking against the floor.
- children gesture or call out as if they want you to restart the activity.
Move to
- some of the more difficult pre-verbal activities (e.g. pp. 85, 107, 119, 133–40.
- activities dealing with imitation (pp. 155–67).
- recognition of sounds (pp. 141–54).

LESS DIFFICULT ACTIVITIES

Children who make no attempt to propel themselves can still benefit from experience of the sense of movement. They can be taken for trips round the room or the playground. Older, more able children may enjoy the responsibility of doing this for you.

Making things happen
Simple mechanical toys

AIM

The children will operate simple mechanical toys of their own accord.

SUITABILITY

The activity is suitable for children who
- reach out to pick up things.
- explore objects by hand and eye.
- do not understand language yet.
- are at Stage 2 (p. 17) of our scheme for the development of communication.

   The activity is not suitable for children who are so profoundly handicapped that they often seem to be asleep.

MATERIALS

Musical boxes made to play by a downward pull on a string.
Musical boxes made to play by turning a simple knob-wind.
Musical boxes which play when the lid is lifted.
Wooden manikins and animals which wave their legs by means of a string-pull.
Jack-in-the-Box.
Pop-up toy.

PROCEDURE

Select a toy which you think the children will like.

   Make sure that they have the ability to make it work — the knob-wind musical box can be difficult.

   Play with the children, showing them how the toy works.

   Encourage any move they make to operate it of their own accord.

   Help them make the required action if necessary.

   Continue to help them for a little, even after they have made their first successful attempt.

TEACHING HINTS

1 Don't stop at one toy. Teach the child to use a variety of them.
2 Talk about the activity to make it more interesting.

3 Look out for signs that a child has copied another child (or an adult) by operating a mechanical toy in an unusual way (e.g. turning the knob-wind of a music box in his teeth). This could indicate better imitative ability (pp. 155–67) than the child has been credited with previously.

Use a diary or day-sheet (p. 281).

MOVING ON

Move on when the children can operate a few simple mechanical toys of their own accord.

Move to activities on imitation (pp. 155–67), recognition of sounds (pp. 141–54), and preparation for words (pp. 176–86).

LESS DIFFICULT ACTIVITIES

If the children do not begin to operate a few toys of their own accord, even with help, return to simpler activities (pp. 121–8).

Understanding the positioning of objects
Watching fast-moving toy cars

AIM

The children will learn that objects can appear in different places.

SUITABILITY

The activity is suitable for children who
- are alert and responsive.
- do not understand language yet.
- are at Stage 2 (p. 17) of our scheme for the development of communication.
  The activity is not suitable for children who
- are so profoundly handicapped that they often seem to be asleep.
- are blind.

MATERIALS

Toy cars, especially those which move quickly because of a motor, a spring, or a flywheel.

PROCEDURE

Make sure you have the children's attention.
    Let the car run across the floor, and encourage the children to watch it.
    If they do watch it, let it run behind a box, chair, or other large object. Encourage any move they make to follow it or look for it when it has gone out of sight.
    Five minutes are sufficient to spend on this activity at any one time.

TEACHING HINTS

1 A car which makes a distinct sound will probably hold the children's interest more powerfully.
2 Join in the activity of looking for the car yourself, to sustain the children's interest.

RECORD-KEEPING

Use a day-sheet (p. 281).

MOVING ON

Move on when children are clearly taking an interest in movement occurring around them, and outside.

Look at other activities concerned with
- positioning and connections (pp. 133–40).
- other non-verbal activities (e.g. p. 85, 103, 111).
- recognition of sounds (pp. 141–54).

LESS DIFFICULT ACTIVITIES

If necessary, bring the children nearer to the path of the car, and use an assistant to turn their heads so that their gaze follows its movement.

Use a car that does not travel too quickly, and do not let it travel all the way across the floor.

Understanding the positioning of objects
Sounds from hidden objects

(Another version of this activity appears on p. 149).

AIM

The children will find a toy by listening for the sound it makes.

SUITABILITY

The activity is suitable for children who
- are responsive.
- explore their surroundings.
- are at Stage 2 (p. 17) of our scheme for the development of communication.
  The activity is not suitable for children who
- have a severe hearing loss.
- are so profoundly handicapped that they often seem to be asleep.

MATERIALS

Musical boxes, small transistor radios, any other clockwork or battery-powered toys which produce a sound.
  Cloth, or cardboard box, under which the toys can be hidden.

PROCEDURE

Switch on the toy after hiding it under the cloth or box. The cloth or box should be near the children if they are hard of hearing or if they do not move about very much.
  Draw their attention to the sound and pretend to look for it. 'Find' it quickly in the early stages of the activity.
  Encourage the children to look for the toy too. Help them as much as they need. Show them that you are pleased when they uncover the toy. Fade out your help as they become better at uncovering the toy.
  Later, begin to hide it in more out-of-the-way locations.

TEACHING HINTS

Don't make the exercise too difficult too quickly. The main thing for the children to learn is that sounds come from a source.

RECORD-KEEPING

Use a day-sheet (p. 281).

MOVING ON

When the children can find sounding objects without difficulty, move to
- pp. 135–40 for other activities concerned with the position of things.
- pp. 107, 123, 129 for harder pre-verbal activities of various kinds.
- pp. 141–54 for exercises on recognition of sounds.

LESS DIFFICULT ACTIVITIES

If the children do not begin to search for hidden, sounding objects, look at
- some of the easier sound-recognition activities (pp. 141–54).
- activities for catching and holding attention (pp. 77–85).

Understanding the positioning of objects
Movement caused by the pull of gravity

AIM

The children will learn that objects will fall or will move downwards when they are not supported.

SUITABILITY

The activity is suitable for children who
● can pick things up with their fingers.
● do not understand language yet.
● are at Stage 2 (p. 17) of our scheme for the development of communication.
  The activity is not suitable for children who are very unresponsive.

MATERIALS

'Slinky' (a coiled spring that 'walks' downstairs).
Plastic people and animals designed to walk down a slope.
Marbles.
Toy cars.
A short plank of wood.
Down Box (p. 199).

PROCEDURE

Let the children see the Slinky toy walking downstairs or down the steps of a chute.
    Let them see other toys slowly rolling down the plank of wood which has been raised at one end to form a slope.
    Let them see toys rolling into the Down Box.
    Encourage any attempt they make to roll the toys of their own accord, or to help you roll them.
    Five to ten minutes of this activity at a time should be sufficient.

TEACHING HINTS

Talk about the activity, and make 'sound-effects' with your voice, to sustain the children's interest in what is going on.

RECORD-KEEPING

Make notes in a diary or use a day-sheet (p. 281).

MOVING ON

Move on when the children take part in any of the activities (or any similar ones in which dropping occurs).
   Look at
- other non-verbal activities (e.g. pp. 107, 123, 129).
- imitation (pp. 155–67).
- understanding of sounds (pp. 141–54).

LESS DIFFICULT ACTIVITIES

If the children show no interest in making or watching objects fall, look at
- activities for helping them to take an interest in moving objects (p. 131).
- activities for developing reaching (pp. 109–12).
- activities for developing their ability to manipulate objects (pp. 87–103).

Understanding the positioning of objects
Building towers

AIM

The children will learn that objects can support each other.

SUITABILITY

The activity is suitable for children who
- can pick things up with their fingers, especially if they can work with both hands.
- are at Stage 2 (p. 17) of our scheme for the development of communication.
  The activity is not suitable for children who are very unresponsive.

MATERIALS

Building-bricks in wood (preferably) or plastic.
Stacking-cups.

PROCEDURE

Help the children to build a tower of three or four bricks.

Talk about the activity to keep up their interest. Don't worry if they cannot build very well in this activity. The aim is to show them that one object can support another.

Encourage any attempt they make to carry out the activity of their own accord.

This activity can last for ten minutes at a time.

TEACHING HINTS

1 Do not use materials which are very awkward for the children to handle. For example, plastic bricks should be avoided if you have wooden ones.
2 Let the children knock down the towers that you build. This helps to prolong interest in the activity.

RECORD-KEEPING

Use a day-sheet (p. 281).

MOVING ON

Move on when the children try to join in the activity of their own accord, especially if they are succeeding.

Look at

- other non-verbal activities (between pp. 77 and 136).
- imitation (pp. 155–67).
- understanding of sounds (pp. 141–54).

LESS DIFFICULT ACTIVITIES

If the children do not begin to show any interest in the activity, look at
- activities to help them reach for things (pp. 109–12).
- activities to catch and hold their attention (pp. 77–84, 131).

Understanding the positioning of objects
Postboxes, pegboards, and formboards

AIM

The children will learn that objects can fit inside each other.

SUITABILITY

The activity is suitable for children who
- can pick things up with their fingers.
- do not understand language yet.
- are at Stage 2 (p. 17) of our scheme for the development of communication.
  The activity is not suitable for children who
- are very unresponsive.
- have very poor concentration.

MATERIALS

Postboxes for shapes.
Pegboards.
Formboards.
Hammer-pegs.
Wooden railway-track.

PROCEDURE

Show the children that the various inserts will fit inside their boards and boxes.

Encourage them to take part and praise any attempts they make.

Help them as necessary. This activity is simply to show that objects can fit inside each other. It is not an exercise in hand-eye co-ordination at this stage.

Ten minutes can be spent on this activity at any one time.

TEACHING HINTS

Most formboards and postboxes are too difficult to be of any use without careful supervision. Encourage any interest the children show in dropping things into containers or sticking things through holes.

RECORD-KEEPING

Keep notes on a day-sheet (p. 281).

MOVING ON

When the children deliberately put objects inside objects and join objects together in their free play, move on to
- other non-verbal activities — there is a wide selection between pages 77 and 138.
- imitation (pp. 155–67).
- recognition of sounds (pp. 141–54).

LESS DIFFICULT ACTIVITIES

If the children do not begin to play at fitting objects into each other, look at more simple ways of manipulating objects (pp. 87–106, 131).

Recognizing and understanding sounds
Outdoor sounds

AIM

The children will become aware of a wide range of sounds in their environment.

SUITABILITY

The activity is suitable for children who
- take an interest in their surroundings.
- do not understand language yet.
- are at Stage 2 (p. 17) of our scheme for the development of communication.
  The activity is not suitable for children who are so profoundly handicapped that they often appear to be asleep.

MATERIALS

None.

PROCEDURE

In this activity you can simply draw the children's attention to sounds that can be heard when you go out for a walk in your neighbourhood.

Birdsong, a lighthouse foghorn, falling rain, the squeal of brakes from a bus, police and fire sirens, the bark of a dog, and the 'green man' Pelican-crossing are all typical examples.

If necessary you can draw the children's attention to the sound, using short sentences such as 'What a noisy bus', 'Hear the bird?', and 'Here's the fire-engine'.

You can also produce outdoor sounds that may interest the children visually as well as aurally. Dropping a stone in a pool and kicking autumn leaves are examples.

TEACHING HINTS

Use short sentences when you are pointing out things to the children. Three or four words to a sentence is long enough.

RECORD-KEEPING
Occasional notes in a diary will be sufficient.

MOVING ON

If the children are clearly interested in the sounds they hear, look at
- harder sound-recognition exercises (pp. 143–54).
- activities for developing thinking (between pp. 77 and 140).
- imitation (pp. 155–67).

LESS DIFFICULT ACTIVITIES

Some children will be so severely handicapped that they will not show any interest in the sounds that can be heard outdoors. All the same, taking them outside may be a pleasurable experience.

Activities for stimulating the sense of hearing of the most profoundly handicapped children appear on pp. 27–40.

Recognizing and understanding sounds
Musical and noise-making toys

AIM

The children will become aware of a wide range of sounds in their environment.

SUITABILITY

The activity is suitable for children who
• take an interest in their surroundings.
• do not understand language yet.
• are at Stage 2 (p. 17) of our scheme for the development of communication.
   The activity is not suitable for children who are so profoundly handicapped that they often appear to be asleep.

MATERIALS

Musical boxes, Christmas mobiles, clockwork vehicles and animals, battery-powered vehicles and animals.

PROCEDURE

Set the toys in motion.
   Imitate the sounds that the toys are making (when this is possible).
   Draw attention to the sound by cupping your hand to your ear and saying 'Listen!' or 'Here it is!' just before you switch it on. If you like, build up an atmosphere of playful suspense before releasing the toy.
   Watch what the children do when the toy has stopped. Do they
• 'tell' you, by becoming agitated, to restart it?
• hand the toy to you?
• try to restart it themselves?
   Show them that you are pleased if they make any of these signs.

TEACHING HINTS

1 The answers to the three questions at the end of 'Procedure' will guide you to the children's most likely level in other pre-verbal activities between pp. 77 and 140.
2 If possible, take your lead from the children. When they pick up one of the toys, join them and discover what sounds it can make.

143

RECORD-KEEPING

Use a diary or day-sheet (p. 281).

MOVING ON

The activities on pp. 145–8 are about the same standard as this one.

If the children are able to make the toys sound of their own accord, keep this activity for recreation. Look for new activities among

- harder sound-recognition activities (pp. 149–54).
- some of the harder activities for developing thinking (e.g. pp. 107, 123, 129).
- imitation (pp. 155–67).

LESS DIFFICULT ACTIVITIES

This activity will be suitable even for children who are very severely handicapped. However, look at the activities for stimulating the sense of hearing (pp. 27–40) if the children show little interest.

Recognizing and understanding sounds
Simple musical instruments

AIM

The children will become aware of a wide range of sounds in their environment.

SUITABILITY

The activity is suitable for children who
● take an interest in their surroundings.
● do not understand language yet.
● are at Stage 2 (p. 17) of our scheme for the development of communication.
   The activity is not suitable for children who are so profoundly handicapped that they often appear to be asleep.

MATERIALS

Drum, tambourine, cymbals, flute, whistle, bottle-xylophone.

PROCEDURE

Explore with the children the variety of sounds which can be made when instruments are sounded.
   Make drums and tambourines sound loudly and quietly by varying the force with which they are hit. Vary the clarity of sound they make — dull with the heel of your hand and sharp with the finger tips; dull and loud at the centre of the skin, sharp and quiet at the rim. Padded drumsticks produce sounds that are different from the sounds produced by wooden ones.
   Show surprise when you 'discover' that one part of a pair of tom-toms produces a higher-pitched note than the other. Similarly, an empty hanging bottle will produce a lower note than a half-full one of the same size. Whistles and flutes can be blown softly or loudly. Cymbals, wood-blocks and castanets produce interesting tone colours. This is principally a 'listening' activity, but encourage any attempt the children make to join in.

TEACHING HINTS

1 If possible, take your lead from the children. When they pick up an instrument, join them, and discover together what sounds it can make.
2 Put your hands over your ears and look frightened when loud noises are

145

made. Cup your hand to your ear to pretend that this will let you hear quiet ones more clearly.

3 If you use a recorder (or other flute that may screech) cover the thumb hole and the highest three finger-holes with insulating tape. That way it produces a more mellow sound.

RECORD-KEEPING

Use a diary or day-sheet (p. 281).

MOVING ON

The activities on pp. 143–8 are about the same standard as this one. If the children begin to join in and play the instruments, keep this activity for recreation. Look for new activities among

- harder sound-recognition activities (pp. 149–54).
- some of the harder activities for developing the powers of thinking (pp. 107, 123, 129).
- imitation (pp. 155–67).

LESS DIFFICULT ACTIVITIES

This activity will be suitable even for children who are very severely handicapped. However, look at the activities for stimulating the sense of hearing (pp. 27–40), if the child shows little interest.

Recognizing and understanding sounds
Sounds from household objects

AIM

The children will become aware of a wide range of sounds in their environment.

SUITABILITY

The activity is suitable for children who
• take an interest in their surroundings.
• do not understand language yet.
• are at Stage 2 (p. 17) of our scheme for the development of communication.
    The activity is not suitable for children who are so profoundly handicapped that they often appear to be asleep.

MATERIALS

Clock, watch, telephone, doorbell, doorknocker, scissors, shoe-brush, lavatory cistern, kitchen sink.

PROCEDURE

In this activity you will simply draw the children's attention to noises that occur around the house or school. Phrases like 'That's the 'phone' or 'Who's that knocking?' can be used to direct their attention as soon as the sound has occurred.
    Encourage the children if they try to produce sounds by manipulating the objects themselves.

TEACHING HINTS

1 Draw the children's attention to the sounds with as few words as possible — three- or four-word sentences are long enough.
2 Watch out for any signs of frustration if the children cannot operate the objects effectively. Divert their attention to something else.
3 If possible, take your lead from the children. When they pick up one of the objects, join them and discover what sounds it can make.

RECORD-KEEPING

Occasional notes in a diary should be sufficient.

MOVING ON

The activities on pp. 143–6 are about the same standard as this one. When the children are exploring the use of everyday objects of their own accord, look for new activities among
- harder sound-recognition activities (pp. 149–54).
- some of the harder activities for developing thinking (pp. 107, 123, 129).
- imitation (pp. 155–67).

LESS DIFFICULT ACTIVITIES

If the children do not begin to take much interest in the sounds that are being produced round about, look at activities for stimulating their hearing (pp. 27–40, 141–6).

Recognizing and understanding sounds
Sounds from hidden objects

AIM

The children will find hidden objects by listening for the sounds they make.

SUITABILITY

The activity is suitable for children who
• take an interest in their surroundings.
• understand little or no language yet.
• have difficulty with 'permanence' (watching and finding) activities on pp. 77–86.
• are at Stage 2 (p. 17) of our scheme for the development of communication.
    The activity is not suitable for children who are so profoundly handicapped that they often seem to be asleep.

MATERIALS

Toys and household objects (such as clocks) which produce a distinctive sound. Screens: large cardboard boxes, pieces of cloth.

PROCEDURE

(a) Make a toy (e.g. a squeaky rubber duck) sound behind the children when they are not looking. Encourage any move they make to turn round and reach for it.

(b) Cut one side from a large cardboard box. Sit in front of the children and make a squeaky toy (or some other object) sound inside the box. Encourage the children to look for it by talking to them and by squeezing the toy occasionally.
Praise any efforts that they make.
    If necessary, give some help. Show them that the box can be lifted. Or let them see part of the sounding object to encourage them to reach for it. If this works, gradually make the object more difficult to find, until it is hidden completely.

(c) Hide objects in various parts of the room. Use objects which are powered by battery or clockwork so that they can produce sounds without you being there to squeeze, strike or blow them. Here are some examples:

149

- a clock with a loud tick.
- an alarm clock.
- a musical box.
- a portable radio or tape-recorder.

Draw the children's attention to the sound and encourage them to look for it. Join them in the search; if necessary, help them so that they find it fairly quickly at first.

Talk about what you are doing to sustain interest.

TEACHING HINTS

1 Use sounding objects which are likely to interest the children.
2 Do not talk too much during the activity — just enough to hold their interest. Sentences of three or four words will be sufficient.
3 If you see signs of frustration or boredom, let the children find the object quickly.
4 Five to ten minutes at a time will be sufficient to spend on this activity.

RECORD-KEEPING

Use a diary or day-sheet (p. 281).

MOVING ON

When the children carry out activity (a), move to activity (b), and from it to activity (c).

Then look at

- other activities for developing recognition of sounds (pp. 141–54).
- some of the harder activities for developing thinking (e.g. pp. 107, 123, 129).
- imitation (pp. 155–67).

LESS DIFFICULT ACTIVITIES

If this activity is too difficult for the children, look at

- activities in which they have to listen rather than react (pp. 141–6).
- activities which will help to catch and hold their attention (pp. 77–84, 131).

Recognizing and understanding sounds
Associating objects with the sounds they produce

AIM

The children will recognize the sound of a familiar object when they hear it on tape.

SUITABILITY

The activity is suitable for children who
- take an interest in their surroundings.
- understand little or no language yet.
- have reached Stage 3 (p. 19) or have advanced well into Stage 2 (p. 17) of our scheme for the development of communication.

The activity is not suitable for children who would have difficulty with the activities on pp. 141–50.

MATERIALS

Tape-recorder.
Musical instruments and other sound-producing objects which the children are able to operate, and whose sounds they like.

PROCEDURE

Make tape-recordings lasting at least 30 seconds of the objects you have decided to use.

Show the children that you want them to sound the first object that appears on the recording. Sound it yourself if that will help.

Stop them after a few seconds and switch on the tape-recorder. Sound the instrument yourself along with the tape-recording. Give the instrument to the children and encourage them to join in.

Rewind the tape, then repeat the activity several times more.

When the children join in the activity with little encouragement, add the recording of another instrument after the recording of the first one. Repeat the process with this instrument.

When the children are happy to sound the second instrument also, return to the tape-recording of the first instrument.

Put both instruments in front of them and switch on the tape-recorder. Encourage the children to join in, and praise them if they pick up the correct instrument. If they do not, give them the correct one and praise them if they then play it.

151

Other instruments can be added as the children's ability increases.

1 Make your first tape-recordings quite lengthy, to save rewinding too often in the course of the activity.
2 Leave a silent gap of a few seconds between the recordings of different instruments on the tape. That will help you find good starting-points more easily when you rewind.
3 Do not rush ahead too quickly with this activity. Five minutes at a time will be enough.

RECORD-KEEPING

A day-sheet (p. 281) would be suitable.

MOVING ON

When the children are able to reach for instruments that they hear on tape, look at
• imitation (pp. 155–67).
• understanding words (pp. 176–86).

LESS DIFFICULT ACTIVITIES

If this activity is too difficult for the children, spend more time on the easier activities of the section (pp. 141–50).

Recognizing and understanding sounds
Associating sounds with models and pictures

AIM

The children will associate pictures and models of real objects, animals, and people with the sounds made by them.

SUITABILITY

The activity is suitable for children who
• look through picture books with an adult.
• play with small models such as farmyard animals and motor cars.
• have little trouble with sound association (p. 151).
• have little trouble with 'Fun sounds' (p. 166).
• seem to understand a few words.
• are far into Stage 2 (p. 17) of our scheme for the development of communication.
   The activity is not suitable for children who take little or no interest in sounds produced by toys, musical instruments, machinery, animals, and other things in their surroundings.

MATERIALS

Pictures, photographs, and models of a variety of common animals.
Photographs of members of the family.
Photographs of the children and adults at school.
Pictures, photographs, and models of vehicles.
Pictures, photographs, and models of common objects (e.g. a telephone) which
   have a distinctive sound.

PROCEDURE

Prepare tape-recordings of voices and sounds which you think will interest the children.
(a) Play the first voice or sound and bring the children's attention to it. Show the children the object, picture, or photograph which has made the sound. Use few words — 'Look!' or 'It's Daddy!' may be enough.
   Show that you are pleased if the children make any signs of recognition, especially if they reach out to the picture or model.
   Switch off the machine.
   Repeat this several times within about five minutes.

153

(b) On subsequent days, introduce new voices or sounds.

Briefly point out the names of the objects, animals, or people. Do not add too many too quickly.

Do not put two or three models or pictures in front of the children and ask them to choose which one is making the sound — that comes later.

(c) Now you can try to see if the children can match picture or model to sound.

Choose the easiest examples you can imagine to give the children the best chance of success. For example, you could have a tape-recording of their mother's voice and photographs of their mother and a police car.

If they get the idea of looking at, pointing to, or reaching for the correct photograph, you can try more pairs of photographs, and later move to three or four.

If they do not get the idea, stay at Stage (b). Give them plenty of opportunity to associate sounds with photographs (pictures and models), but do not confuse them by asking them to make a choice just yet.

TEACHING HINTS

1 Polaroid or Kodak instant cameras are an easy means of collecting photographs for this activity.
2 Be honest about the quality of your tape-recording. Discard examples which are not good enough, and try again. The BBC markets a wide range of sound effects tapes.
3 Make your first tape-recordings (for Stages (a) and (b)) quite lengthy. This will save a lot of rewinding. The examples can be shorter at Stage (c).
4 Line-drawings, even outline-drawings, may be clearer to understand than some photographs or pictures. Experiment with them if the children do not seem to understand ordinary pictures or photographs. This applies with partially sighted children too.

RECORD-KEEPING

Notes in a diary may be sufficient, though a day-sheet would probably be better.

MOVING ON

Children who tackle Stage (c) of this activity successfully can move to
• imitation (pp. 155–67).
• understanding words (pp. 176–90).

LESS DIFFICULT ACTIVITIES

If this activity is too difficult for the children, spend more time on the easier activities of the section (pp. 141–52).

Imitating actions
Simple actions with objects

AIM

The children will copy actions that they see other people perform.

SUITABILITY

The activity is suitable for children who
- pick up objects and examine them closely.
- knock objects together, or take part in some other simple kinds of play.
- may already have copied the actions of another child.
- have reached Stage 3 (p. 19) of our scheme for the development of communication.

  The activity is not suitable for children who
- do not pick up objects of their own accord.
- are only just beginning to reach out for objects.

MATERIALS

Various small objects found in most classrooms. Specific examples are provided in 'Procedure'.

PROCEDURE

Carry out the activity when the children are in a co-operative mood.

Try to make it seem like a game, not a test.

Five to ten minutes at a time will be sufficient to spend on this activity.

Show the children the activity you want them to copy, and encourage them to take part.

Here are some examples:

Squeaky toy	: squeeze the toy by hand.
Cup and bead	: drop the bead into the cup.
Handbell	: shake it.
Building-bricks	: stack them; knock a tower over.
Ball	: push/roll it along the floor or table.
Rubber ring	: throw.
Stacking-cups	: put one inside the other.
Crinkly paper	: crumple into a ball inside two hands.

Hat   : put on head.
Cup and spoon : stir.
Toy car   : push along.
Flower and vase: put flower in vase
Football   : kick.

TEACHING HINTS

1 If the children do not join in, they may simply be bored or may not like the
   activity. However, imitation may just be too difficult for them; this would
   probably be the case if you found they could not tackle the harder pre-verbal
   exercises for developing thinking (e.g. pp. 107, 123, 129).
2 If the children show a liking for any materials in particular, make up imitation
   activities of your own, using these materials.
3 Guide the children's hands through the activity if you think this will help them
   to get the idea more quickly.

RECORD-KEEPING

Use a diary or day-sheet (p. 281).

MOVING ON

If the children can carry out this activity, look at
● make-believe play (pp. 168–75).
● imitation of visible and invisible gestures (pp. 157–60).
● imitation of sounds (pp. 164–7).
● understanding words (pp. 176–90).
● music and movement (p. 161).

LESS DIFFICULT ACTIVITIES

If the children are unable to imitate actions which are carried out on objects,
discover if they can imitate visible or invisible actions (pp. 157–60). If these are
too difficult, look at some of the other non-verbal activities (e.g. pp. 83, 97, 125).

Imitating actions
Visible actions

AIM

The children will copy an action that they can see themselves perform.

SUITABILITY

The activity is suitable for children who
- pick up objects and examine them closely.
- knock objects together, or take part in some other simple sorts of play.
- have reached Stage 3 (p. 19) of our scheme for the development of communication.
  The activity is not suitable for children who
- do not pick up objects of their own accord.
- are only just beginning to reach out for objects.

MATERIALS

None.

PROCEDURE

Take note of any gestures or movements which the children make of their own accord, and which they can see when they have carried them out. For example, waving, clapping, and sitting cross-legged are actions which they can see.
(a) At a time when they are not carrying out any of these actions, perform one in front of them several times and encourage them to take part.
    If necessary, give them some help to show that you want them to copy you — for example, move their limbs into position. Show them that you are pleased when the imitation has been made.
(b) When the children can successfully imitate visible gestures and movements which you have seen them make, try with ones which you have not seen them make before. Here are some possible examples:
- slapping one's own thighs.
- rubbing hands together.
- finger on nose.
- opening and closing fist.
- bending and stretching index finger.
- drumming hands on table.

TEACHING HINTS

1 Carry out this activity when the children are in a co-operative mood. If possible, avoid seating them on the opposite side of a table from yourself, and working through the activity as if it were a test.
2 Do not worry if the children do not copy you to order. They may see no point in the activity. However, look out for signs in their free play which suggest that they have been watching, copying, and learning from the behaviour of adults and other children.

RECORD-KEEPING

Use a diary or day sheet (p. 281).

MOVING ON

If the children copy unfamiliar gestures and movements easily, look at
• imitation of invisible actions (p. 159).
• make-believe play (pp. 168–75).
• imitation of sounds (pp. 164–7).
• understanding words (pp. 176–90).
• 'Music and movement' (p. 161).

LESS DIFFICULT ACTIVITIES

If the children do not join in this type of imitative activity, they may simply be not very interested by it. You could check this by watching them at 'Music and movement' (p. 161) or simple make-believe play.

However if they show no signs at all of being able to imitate, return to easier non-verbal activities (e.g. pp. 85, 97, and 125).

Imitating actions
Invisible actions

AIM

The children will copy an action that they cannot see themselves perform.

SUITABILITY

The activity is suitable for children who
- pick up objects and examine them closely.
- knock objects together, or take part in some other simple kinds of play.
- may already have copied the actions of another child.
- have reached Stage 3 (p. 19) of our scheme for the development of communication.
  The activity is not suitable for children who
- do not pick up objects of their own accord.
- are only just beginning to reach out for objects.

MATERIALS

None.

PROCEDURE

Take note of any gestures or movements which the children make of their own accord, and which they cannot see when they are carrying them out. Scratching the top of their head and pulling their ear-lobe are two examples.
(a) At a time when they are not carrying out one of these actions, perform it in front of them several times, and encourage them to take part.

If necessary, give them some help to show them that you want them to copy you — for example, move their limbs into position. Show them that you are pleased when the imitation has been made.
(b) When the children can successfully imitate invisible gestures and movements which you have seen them make, try them with ones which you have not seem them make before. Here are some possible examples:
- patting the back of their head.
- blinking.
- opening and shutting the mouth.
- wrinkling the nose.

TEACHING HINTS

1 Carry out this activity when the children are in a co-operative mood. If possible, avoid seating them on the opposite side of a table from yourself, and working through the activity as if it were a test.
2 Do not worry if the children do not copy you to order. They may see no point in the activity. However, look out for signs in their free play which suggest that they have been watching, copying, and learning from the behaviour of adults and other children.

RECORD-KEEPING

Use a diary or day-sheet (p. 281).

MOVING ON

If the children copy unfamiliar invisible gestures and movements easily, look at
• make-believe play (pp. 168–75).
• imitation of sounds (pp. 164–7).
• understanding words (pp. 176–90).
• 'Music and movement' (p. 161).

LESS DIFFICULT ACTIVITIES

If the children do not join in this type of imitative activity, they may not be very interested in it. You could check this by watching them at 'Music and movement' (p. 161), or simple make-believe play. Look also at imitation of visible actions (p. 157) as that may be slightly easier.

However, if they show no signs at all of being able to imitate, return to easier non-verbal activities (e.g. pp. 85, 97, 125).

Imitating actions
Music and movement

AIM

The children will imitate actions of other people.
The children will learn to connect an action with a sound which triggers it off.
The children will learn to connect words of command with actions.

SUITABILITY

The activity is suitable for children who
● are able to walk.
● explore their surroundings.
● have been seen carrying out actions which they have copied from other people.
● are at least at Stage 3 (p. 19) of our scheme for the development of communication.

　　With adaptations it can also be suitable for children who have restricted mobility as a result of severe physical handicap.

MATERIALS

Piano or tape-recorder.

PROCEDURE

Make a list of actions which the children you work with could carry out to music.
The following list will act as a guide:
● giant, slow steps.
● little steps.
● tip-toe walking.
● crawling.
● running.
● flying (arm-flapping like a bird).
● see-saw (with a partner).
● clapping hands.
● nodding head.
● yawning and stretching.
● marching.
● rolling over and over on the floor.
● growing smaller and smaller.
● falling down.

- growing bigger and bigger.
- standing straight up.
- bouncing.

Select a group of actions for about ten to fifteen minutes of group activity and match each activity to a different tune or musical sound. Tape-record this music if you cannot play the piano. 'Music and Movement' is a useful group activity to have every day, but try to fit it in at least twice a week.

If necessary, help the children to perform the actions of the activity and praise them by name when you see signs of improvement. Physically handicapped children may each require a helper during 'Music and Movement'. Some schools have sufficient staff to allow this, but others could use parents, voluntary workers, or community-service pupils from local secondary schools.

TEACHING HINTS

1 The *Apusskidu* and *Okki-tokki-unga* collections (Harrop 1976 and Harrop, Blakeley, and Gadsby 1975) are good sources of tunes for 'Music and Movement'.
2 If you use a tape-recorder, be honest about the quality of the recording. Make fresh recordings if your first efforts are unsatisfactory.
3 A chord of A, C sharp, F natural, is a good sharp sound for 'freeze' or 'fall down'.
4 Sing along with the music; some children respond better to song than to ordinary speech.
5 Emphasize the command words, using very short sentences — one word long when possible.

RECORD-KEEPING

You cannot keep notes on 'Music and Movement' for an entire class. Note any unusual happenings in the diaries of individual children.

MOVING ON

Children who have no trouble with 'Music and Movement' are ready for
- understanding words (pp. 176–90).
- first words (pp. 191–211).
and perhaps for
- connected speech (p. 225–37).
- developing understanding (pp. 212–24).

LESS DIFFICULT ACTIVITIES

If the children cannot imitate the actions you want, individual activities for developing imitation may be more suitable (pp. 155–60).

However, continue to let them take part in 'Music and Movement', as they will probably enjoy the company of the other children, and may be encouraged to join in as best they can.

Imitating vocal sounds
Increasing the child's range of sounds

AIM

The children will increase the range of vocal sounds they produce.
The children will notice changes in the vocal sounds of other people.

SUITABILITY

The activity is suitable for children who
- babble.
- make any other vocal sounds which are not words.
- have advanced well into Stage 2 (p. 17) of our scheme for the development of communication.
  The activity is not suitable for children who
- take very little interest in their surroundings.
- do not make vocal sounds.

MATERIALS

No special materials, though a hair-drier hose or a Tok-Bak (ESA Special Education Catalogue) could be useful.

PROCEDURE

Make a note of any babbling or other vocal sounds which the children have been heard making.

Carry out the activity when the children are producing sounds. Show them you are pleased that they are babbling and encourage them to produce more. Let them use a hair-drier hose, Tok-Bak, or some other amplifier if you think this will help.

Babble back to them the sound they are making. Note whether they
- ignore you.
- stop, and look quizzically.
- carry on babbling.
- babble at a greater rate.

Babble one of their other sounds on another occasion when they are babbling. Note the effect. Note especially if
- they stop, and look quizzically.
- change to make the sound you are making.

On another occasion, interrupt and babble a sound they have not been heard making. Note the effect.

Finally, respond to their babbling with other types of variation. For example:
- alter the pitch at which you babble.
- alter the length of your babbling.
- babble strings of mixed up sounds (including real words).

TEACHING HINTS

Do not be surprised if the children stop babbling when you start. Many children prefer to babble when they are on their own instead of in company.

RECORD-KEEPING

Keep notes in a diary or a day-sheet (p. 281).

MOVING ON

If you hear the children make definite changes towards the babble-sounds you are making, look at
- 'Fun sounds' (p. 166).
- the earliest kinds of make-believe play (pp. 168–71).
- understanding words (pp. 176–86).

LESS DIFFICULT ACTIVITIES

If the children do not imitate sounds, encourage them to produce any vocal sounds of their own. That will give you something to build on later.

If they produce no vocal sounds at all, check with a speech therapist, doctor, or audiologist in case there is a physical cause for this problem. If there is no physical cause, make sure that the children are being encouraged to take an interest in sounds. Look also at the notes on withdrawn children (p. 267) and on children who have difficulty in forming relationships (p. 269).

Imitating vocal sounds
Fun sounds

AIM

The children will imitate sounds made by an adult.

SUITABILITY

The activity is suitable for children who
- produce a wide range of vocal sounds.
- appear interested in vocal sounds made by other people.
- may have been heard producing an imitation of words or sounds made by someone else, or an animal or a piece of machinery.
- have reached Stage 3 (p. 19) of our scheme for the development of communication.

  The activity is not suitable for children who
- cannot be encouraged to produce vocal sounds.
- do not inspect objects closely or manipulate them.

MATERIALS

Home-made 'fun sound' booklets (collect pictures of objects and animals which make distinctive sounds — staple the pictures into booklets of ten to fifteen pages).

Model animals and sound-producing objects.

PROCEDURE

Choose a suitable set of pictures or models of things that produce sounds. The answers to the following questions may help your choice:

What objects do the children recognize when they are presented in pictures and photographs, or in models?
What sounds are likely to interest or amuse them?
What sounds are easy for them to make?

Staple or tape your collection of pictures into a booklet.
Begin by treating it as you would any story book.
Sit with one or two children and talk about the pictures to them.
Do not worry about getting a response at first, but show the children that you are pleased if you do.
Emphasize the sounds the objects make; try to make the children smile or

laugh when you do. The better you act, the greater is the chance that they will join in.

Here is a sample script for three pictures: a sheep, the green man on a Pelican-crossing, a dog.

Note the short statements and the absence of questions.

Picture 1 Here's the sheep. Sheep says 'Baa'. (Repeat 'Baa' as often as you and the children like.)
Picture 2 Here's the green man [figure in the Pelican-crossing]. Green man says 'Pee-pee-pee-pee-pee-pee'. (Repeat, as before.)
Picture 3 Here's the doggy. Doggy says 'Bow-wow'. (Repeat, as before.)

When the children become responsive, change your script by waiting for a second before giving the 'fun sound'. Encourage any effort the children make to move their lips or make a sound.

Later you can encourage them to look at your lips and move nearer to making the sounds you want. If necessary, move their lips to a better position with your fingers.

TEACHING HINTS

1 If possible, give the children opportunities to see the objects which produce the fun sounds in real life.
2 Keep the 'fun sounds' booklets and models special by storing them away when they are not in use.

RECORD-KEEPING

Use a day-sheet (p. 281) for keeping notes on progress.

MOVING ON

Children who make good imitations of fun sounds are ready for
• understanding words (pp. 176–90).
• first words (p. 191–211).

LESS DIFFICULT ACTIVITIES

If the children do not imitate sounds, encourage them to produce any vocal sounds of their own. That will give you something to build on later.

If they produce no vocal sounds at all, check with a speech therapist, doctor, or audiologist in case there is a physical cause for this problem. If there is no physical cause, make sure that the children are being encouraged to take an interest in sounds. Look also at the notes on withdrawn children (p. 267) and on children who have difficulty in forming relationships (p. 269).

Make-believe play
Everyday activities

AIM

The children will pretend to drink from a cup, comb their hair, wash their face, or carry out some other everyday action.

SUITABILITY

The activity is suitable for children who
- show signs of understanding some words.
- can easily carry out the activities on pp. 155–60.
- have reached at least Stage 3 (p. 19) of our scheme for the development of communication.

    The activity is not suitable for children who
- do not pick up objects and examine them.
- have not played with objects by squeezing, pulling, patting, or otherwise manipulating them.

MATERIALS

Cutlery and crockery (real or model).
Combs, brushes, face-cloths, sponges.
Dolls and soft toys.

PROCEDURE

Try to use this as an activity for a small group of children, although it is also suitable for a single child.

Take the children's lead if possible. For example, if they are playing with a doll's tea-set, join them and pretend to 'drink' from a cup. Encourage them to do the same. Encourage them also if they want to take the activity further and pretend to pour from a tea-pot into the cup.

One step beyond this is pretending to feed dolls and other soft toys. Combing hair and washing faces are similar activities worth encouraging too.

TEACHING HINTS

1 Do not try to rush the children into more difficult types of make-believe too soon. Take the lead from them. 'Feeding' a Teddy bear may make very little

sense to them, even though they are quite happy to pretend to drink from a cup themselves or to make you pretend to drink.

2 Look at p. 172 for some brief advice on the level of difficulty of make-believe activities. See McConkey and Jeffree (1981) and the PIP Charts (Jeffree and McConkey 1976b) for more detailed advice.

RECORD-KEEPING

Use a diary or day-sheet (p. 281).

MOVING ON

When the children are clearly taking part in make-believe play, look at
- recognition of sounds (pp. 149–54).
- imitation (pp. 155–67).
- understanding words (pp. 176–86).

If the children bring a cup to you, indicating that they want to drink (or if they perform some similar action), look at
- understanding words (pp. 176–90).
- first words (pp. 191–202).

LESS DIFFICULT ACTIVITIES

Make-believe is quite an advanced sort of play. If the children do not join in, look at activities concerned with imitating actions (pp. 155–63) and handling objects (e.g. pp. 107, 123).

Make-believe play
Dressing up

AIM

The children will dress up in adult clothing. Much later, they will pretend to be a specific adult such as a nurse or policeman.

SUITABILITY

The activity is suitable for children who
- show signs of understanding some words.
- can easily carry out the activities on pp. 155–60.
- are at least at Stage 3 (p. 19) of our scheme of communication.
  The activity is not suitable for children who
- do not pick up objects and examine them.
- have not played with objects by squeezing, pulling, patting, or otherwise manipulating them.

MATERIALS

Adults' clothing.
Fancy-dress outfits (e.g. cowboy, police).
Hats.
Handbags.

PROCEDURE

Encourage the children to join in when other children in the group are playing at dressing up.

Children often come out of their shell when they are 'disguised' in clothes which are not their own. Take your lead from the children and pay attention if they start giving orders by pointing to things and calling out (without the use of words).

Try to guess what they mean, and behave as if that was what they said. Note their reaction.

TEACHING HINTS

1 This activity can be developed into simple drama. When the children are able to imitate well, they may want to act the part of a policeman, bus-driver, or

dinner-attendant. Encourage this when you see it beginning.

2 For more detailed advice on drama, see McClintock (1984).

RECORD-KEEPING

Occasional notes in a diary should be sufficient.

MOVING ON

Dressing up for make-believe play will always be useful, even when the children are able to speak.

When the children enjoy this activity you should also be working at

• understanding words (pp. 176–90).
• first words (pp. 191–202).

LESS DIFFICULT ACTIVITIES

Make-believe is quite an advanced form of play. If the children do not join in, look at the slightly easier activity on p. 168. If this is still too hard, look at activities concerned with imitation of actions (pp. 155–63).

Make-believe play
Dolls and other models come to life

AIM

The children will play with dolls and soft toys as if they were real people or animals.

SUITABILITY

The activity is suitable for children who
- show signs of understanding some words.
- can easily carry out the activities on pp. 155–60.
- are at least at Stage 3 (p. 19) of our scheme of communication.
  The activity is not suitable for children who
- do not pick up objects and examine them.
- have not played with objects by squeezing, pulling, patting, or otherwise manipulating them.

MATERIALS

Dolls (including Action Man) and other soft toys.
Self-care objects: combs, brushes, face-cloths, etc.
Table-ware: tea-sets, cutlery.
Doll's house and furniture.
Cardboard boxes.

PROCEDURE

This activity can be carried out with one child or with one or two children.

Decide which of the stages in the following list is the level at which the child is playing just now, and make up play activities at about that level. Start with 1, the easiest level, if you are not sure that the child is ready for make-believe play.
1 Hugging or kissing a doll or Teddy bear.
2 Giving the doll a drink from a cup. Feeding it with a biscuit. Combing its hair. Bathing it. Undressing it.
3 Working through a sequence of make-believe activities, e.g. bathing (undressing, bathing, drying, and dressing); putting to bed (undressing, putting in bed, covering up, kissing goodnight).
4 Making doll act like a real person, e.g. making it hold up and drink from a cup.
5 Working through a long sequence of different activities, e.g. feeding, then

washing, then putting to bed.
6 Playing with miniature people in doll's house.

1 If possible, let the children take the lead in starting this activity.
2 View 'Learning to pretend' (McConkey 1984) for further advice on make-believe play.

RECORD-KEEPING

Notes in a diary will be sufficient, but you could use a day-sheet (see p. 281) if you think it necessary to keep a more detailed record.

MOVING ON

Move through the six levels above as the child's ability grows.
  For levels 1–3, look also at
• recognition of sounds (pp. 141–54).
• imitation (pp. 155–67).
• understanding words (pp. 176–86).
  For levels 4–6, look at
• imitation (pp. 155–67).
• understanding words (pp. 176–90).
• first words (pp. 191–202).

LESS DIFFICULT ACTIVITIES

Make-believe is quite an advanced form of play. If a child does not join in, look at the easier activities on pp. 168–71. If these are still too hard, look at activities concerned with imitation of actions (pp. 155–63) and handling objects (e.g. pp. 107, 123.

Make-believe play
Cardboard-box vehicles

AIM

The children will use a cardboard box as if it were a car, a bed, or some other object.

SUITABILITY

The activity is suitable for children who
- show signs of understanding some words.
- play with toys (e.g. cars, games, and dolls) as if they were real or alive.
- are at least at Stage 3 (p. 19) of our scheme for the development of communication.
    The activity is not suitable for children who have not been seen taking part in any pretend play.

MATERIALS

Large cardboard boxes.

PROCEDURE

Work with one child or a small group.
    Encourage the children to see imaginative possibilities for using boxes. Here are some examples:
1 Seat children in the box and push them, pretending that the box is a car. Make engine noises, and talk about what you are doing to add interest.
2 Turn a cardboard box upside-down, cut a hole in one end, and use it as a garage. Make engine noises as cars are driven into it.
3 Use a cardboard box as a doll's bed. Encourage the child to lay the doll in it, and cover it with a cloth.

TEACHING HINTS

If possible, let the children take the lead in starting the activity, for example, by picking up a doll.

RECORD-KEEPING

Notes in a diary should be adequate. A day-sheet could also be used if you require more detailed records.

MOVING ON

Move on if a child spontaneously uses cardboard boxes as if they were other objects.

Look at
- the more difficult imitation exercises (between pp. 155 and 167).
- recognition of sounds (pp. 151–4).
- understanding words (pp. 176–90).
- first words (pp. 191–202).

LESS DIFFICULT ACTIVITIES

Make-believe is not a simple form of play. If this activity seems to have little meaning for a child, some of the earlier make-believe activities (pp. 168–73) and the activities dealing with imitation of actions (pp. 155–63) might be tried.

Understanding words
Introducing nouns and pronouns

AIM

The children will understand some nouns and pronouns.

SUITABILITY

The activity is suitable for children who
- can understand some spoken words already.
- can follow simple commands such as 'Stop it', or 'Come here' (with or without gestures being used).
- take notice when they hear their names being spoken in the conversation of adults.
- recognize the name of the occasional person or object.
- are at Stage 3 (p. 19) of our scheme for the development of communication.
    The activity is not suitable for children who are unable to tackle the harder activities for developing recognition of sounds (pp. 149–54).

MATERIALS

Photographs and pictures of people, animals, and objects. The ESA catalogue has
    a good selection.
Polaroid camera — for obtaining special photographs quickly.
Models of animals, and objects.
Toy furniture, with or without doll's house.
Dolls, Action Man, soft toys, and puppets.
A variety of boxes or hiding toys.
A box with a trap door (for sudden disappearances).

PROCEDURE

Your job now may seem rather difficult as you will have no check on how well your teaching is progressing for some little time. Your job is to present the target words to the children in as many ways as possible but *at this stage you must resist the temptation to test the children's acquisition of what you have been trying to teach.*

1 Choose approximately four target words from table 6. Any words will do, but try to select ones which the children do not seem to understand, and ones which are likely to be interesting.

Table 6 Target words for noun/pronoun comprehension

Personal	
Names	Child's own name, Mummy, Daddy, baby, the names of one or two members of staff, names of brothers or sisters, me
Body parts	Eye, nose, toe, teeth, hair, hand, mouth
Clothing	Shoe, button, coat, hat, socks
In the house and school	
Food	Biscuit, drink (or milk or tea or juice), toast, banana, cake, peas, potatoes, mince
Furniture and utensils	Cloth, bath, door, spoon, bed, chair, house
Toys	Ball, book, Teddy, bubbles, brick (block), balloon, dolly
Outdoors	
Animals	Bird, dog, horse, cow, cat, fish, duck
Garden and countryside	Tree, see-saw, flowers, swings
Vehicles	Car, bike, bus, train, lorry, plane

2 Present the target words to the child in as many ways as possible. Here are some examples using the target word 'dog' or 'doggie':

(i) Talk about real dogs which the children can see out-of-doors or on television.

(ii) Make use of any interest which the children have shown in the dog spontaneously.

(iii) Photographs and pictures

(a) Large individual pictures. These are useful for catching attention initially.

(b) Home-made picture books. Collect pictures and photographs of dogs, and glue them to sheets of paper which can be folded into booklets. These booklets can be dismantled and reassembled to include pictures of other objects, as the child's target vocabulary increases.

(c) Commercially produced picture books. You *may* find picture books devoted entirely to dogs, but if not, use general picture books in which they occur only occasionally. This introduces surprise into the activity.

(d) Picture cubes. Glue photographs or pictures of dogs to the sides of wooden, polystyrene, or cardboard cubes of various sizes. Roll them on the floor or turn them over and over by hand; up to six different people or objects can be displayed on each cube.

(e) 35 mm transparencies. Show these in a battery-powered hand viewer. Include a picture of the child's own dog if there is one at home.

(iv) Models and other toys

Model dogs can appear in toy farmyards; sit on the chairs and beds of toy furniture; go for a ride in toy cars; hide under cardboard boxes; fall down into boxes with trapdoors.

TEACHING HINTS

1 Use the target words often during individual teaching.

2 Keep your sentences short.
3 Speak in statements rather than questions or demands. For example, 'Here comes doggie' rather than 'Where's doggie?' or 'Show me doggie'. You are showing the children something, not testing them.
4 If possible, let the children take the initiative in starting the activity. Place the pictures (toys, etc.) near them and, if they pick them up, begin talking about them.
5 Store your individual teaching materials away from everyday classroom equipment. This will keep them special and interesting.
6 Give up gracefully if the child is having a bad day (or week!). If you persist, the child may be very difficult to interest on later occasions.
7 Keep your 'lessons' short. Stop before the child loses interest. Five minutes of individual teaching may be more than enough.

RECORD-KEEPING

Note the target words you have been teaching in a diary or day-sheet (p. 281).

MOVING ON

After a week or so try to find out how well the children are understanding the target words — use the activity on p. 187 to do this. Lengthen or shorten the period of one week, depending on the child's success.

Replace words which the children now understand with new ones from the list (or from your imagination).

The 'First Words' scheme (Gillham 1979) will help to consolidate achievements at this level.

LESS DIFFICULT ACTIVITIES

It is difficult to tell when this activity is too advanced for children — you do not really know until you try to discover how well they have understood the target words. The activity on p. 187 will tell you this.

If they make little progress, return to some of the harder activities for developing recognition of sounds (e.g., pp. 149–54).

Understanding words
Introducing action words

AIM

The child will understand verbs and prepositions which describe action.

SUITABILITY

The activity is suitable for children who
- can understand some spoken words already.
- can follow simple commands such as 'Stop it' or 'Come here' (with or without gestures being used).
- take notice when they hear their names being spoken in the conversation of adults.
- recognize the names of the occasional person or object.
- are at Stage 3 (p. 19) of our scheme for the development of communication.

The activity is not suitable for children who are unable to tackle the harder activities for developing recognition of sounds (e.g. pp. 149–54).

MATERIALS

Photographs and pictures of people, animals, and objects. The ESA Special Education Catalogue has a good selection.
Polaroid camera — for obtaining special photographs quickly.
Models of animals and objects. Toy furniture, with or without doll's house.
Dolls, Action Man, soft toys, and puppets.
A variety of boxes for hiding toys.
A box with a trap door (for sudden disappearances).
Some sturdy apparatus — chairs, benches, boxes — and cushioned matting for acting out the meaning of words.

PROCEDURE

1 Choose one or two target words from the following list:

   down, gone, bang, sit, up, walk, all gone, come, carry, go, bring, give, jump, kick, splash, shut, throw, look.

   Choose words which are likely to interest the children. Add any others which may be successful.

179

2 Present the words in a variety of ways. Here are some examples using the word "up".

    (a) *Acting on objects* Say 'Up' when you lift objects on to a table, chair, or counter. A classroom shop gives a good opportunity for using it: lay a number of tins and boxes on the floor, then lift them to the counter (getting the child to help you), saying, 'Cheese up', 'Beans up', etc.

    (b) *Spontaneous activity by the children* Take advantage of these situations. For example, say something like 'You're high up!' if the child climbs the steps of the chute.

    (c) *Photographs and pictures* Make an 'up' scrapbook which contains pictures of objects, animals, and people which are clearly above some other object, or are up in the air.

    (d) *Models and toys* A small-scale version of (a) and (b) above: dolls' houses, toy farmyards, model garages, and sand-trays present many opportunities for the use of 'up' and other target words.

TEACHING HINTS

1 Use the target words often during individual teaching.
2 Keep your sentences short.
3 Speak in statements rather than questions or demands. For example, 'Doggie's jumping up' rather than 'Is the doggie up?' or 'Show me up'. You are showing the children something, not testing them.
4 If possible, let the children take the initiative in starting the activity. Place the pictures (toys, etc.) near them and, if they pick them up, begin talking about them.
5 Store your individual teaching materials away from everyday classroom equipment. This will keep them special and interesting.
6 Give up gracefully if the children are having a bad day (or week!). If you persist, the children may be very difficult to interest on later occasions.
7 Keep your 'lessons' short. Stop before the children lose interest. Five minutes of individual teaching may be more than enough.

RECORD-KEEPING

Note the target words you have been teaching in a diary or day-sheet (p. 281).

MOVING ON

After a week or so try to find out how well the children understand the target words — use the activity on p. 189 to do this. Lengthen or shorten the period of one week, depending on the children's success.

Replace words which the children now understand with new ones from the list (or from your imagination). The 'First Words' scheme (Gillham 1979) will help to consolidate achievements at this level.

LESS DIFFICULT ACTIVITIES

It is difficult to tell when this activity is too advanced for the children — you do not really know until you try to discover how well they have understood the target words. The activity on p. 187 will tell you this.

If they make little progress, return to some of the harder activities for developing recognition of sounds (e.g. pp. 149–54).

Understanding words
Introducing social vocabulary

AIM

The children will understand elementary social vocabulary.

SUITABILITY

The activity is suitable for children who
- can understand some spoken words already.
- can follow simple commands such as 'Stop it' or 'Come here' (with or without gestures being used).
- take notice when they hear their names being spoken in the conversation of adults.
- recognize the names of the occasional person or object.
- are at Stage 3 (p. 19) of our scheme for the development of communication.
  The activity is not suitable for children who are unable to tackle the harder activities for developing recognition of sounds (e.g. pp. 149–54).

MATERIALS

Photographs and pictures of people, animals, and objects. The ESA Special Education Catalogue has a good selection.
Polaroid camera — for obtaining special photographs quickly.
Models of animals and objects. Toy furniture, with or without doll's house.
Dolls, Action Man, soft toys, and puppets.
A variety of boxes for hiding toys.
A box with a trap door (for sudden disappearances).
Some sturdy apparatus — chairs, benches, boxes — and cushioned matting for acting out the meaning of words.

PROCEDURE

1 Select one or two target words from the following list:

   bye-bye, hello, ta, thank you, please, no, yes, night-night.

2 Here are some suggestions for bringing attention to the word 'bye-bye'.
   (a) *Acting on objects* Make toys vanish by hiding them under containers, by letting them fall into trapdoor boxes, or by covering them with a piece of cloth. Say 'Bye-bye [dolly, dog, car, etc.]', as the object vanishes. When possible, wave 'bye-bye' at the same time.

(b) *Unpredictable opportunities* Make a point of saying 'Bye-bye' when children or adults leave the room. Wave 'Bye-bye' also. When possible, take the child's hand and make it wave when you say 'Bye-bye'.

TEACHING HINTS

1 Use the target words often during individual teaching.
2 Keep your sentences short.
3 Speak in statements rather than questions or demands. For example, 'Bye-bye car, bye-bye bus' rather than 'Can you wave bye-bye?' or 'Show me bye-bye'. You are showing the children something, not testing them.
4 If possible, let the children take the initiative in starting the activity. Place the pictures (toys, etc.) near them and, if they pick them up, begin talking about them.
5 Store your individual teaching materials away from everyday classroom equipment. This will keep them special and interesting.
6 Give up gracefully if the children are having a bad day (or week!). If you persist, the children may be very difficult to interest on later occasions.
7 Keep your 'lessons' short. Stop before the children lose interest. Five minutes of individual teaching may be more than enough.

RECORD-KEEPING

Note the target words you have been teaching in a diary or day-sheet (p. 281).

MOVING ON

After a week or so try to find out how well the children are understanding the target words — use the activity on p. 187 to do this. Lengthen or shorten the period of one week, depending on the children's success.

Replace words which the children now understand with new ones from the list (or from your imagination).

The 'First Words' scheme (Gillham 1979) will help to consolidate achievements at this level.

LESS DIFFICULT ACTIVITIES

It is difficult to tell when this activity is too advanced for children — you do not really know until you try to discover how well they have understood the target words. The activity on p. 187 will tell you this.

If they make little progress, return to some of the harder activities for developing recognition of sounds (e.g. pp. 149–54).

Understanding words
Introducing words which describe objects and events

AIM

The children will understand some words which modify meaning. This group includes adjectives, adverbs, and some prepositions. Usually, they will describe a person, object, action, or position.

SUITABILITY

The activity is suitable for children who
- can understand some spoken words already.
- can follow simple commands such as 'Stop it' or 'Come here' (with or without gestures being used).
- take notice when they hear their names being spoken in the conversation of adults.
- recognize the names of the occasional person or object.
- are at Stage 3 (p. 19) of our scheme for the development of communication.
   The activity is not suitable for children who are unable to tackle the harder activities for developing recognition of sounds (e.g. pp. 149–54).

MATERIALS

Photographs and pictures of people, animals, and objects. The ESA Special Education Catalogue has a good selection.
Polaroid camera — for obtaining special photographs quickly.
Models of animals and objects. Toy furniture, with or without a doll's house.
Dolls, Action Man, soft toys, and puppets.
A variety of boxes for hiding toys.
A box with a trapdoor (for sudden disappearances).
Some sturdy apparatus — chairs, benches, boxes — and cushioned matting for acting out the meaning of the words.

PROCEDURE

1 Select one or two target words from the following list:

   hot, more, where, again, outside, there, dirty, noisy, high, my, bad, big, cold, mine, nice, on, wet, naughty.

2 Here are some ways of presenting the modifying word 'wet'.
  (a) *Acting on objects* Toys, paper and cloth can all be made wet by dropping them in a water-tray or sink. There is a very good chance children will join in this activity of their own accord. Tell them about the change in the object with simple sentences such as 'It's all wet', 'Dolly's got wet', etc.
  (b) *Acting on the child* Tell the children something like 'You're all wet' if they get caught in the rain. Tell them their hands are wet when they have been playing in the water-tray.
  (c) *Unpredictable opportunities* Accidents and the weather result in objects, animals, and people becoming wet. Tell the children about it when these opportunities arise.
  (d) *Photographs and pictures* Make a 'wet' scrapbook containing pictures of objects, animals, and people who have become wet by the rain, falling in pools, etc.

In (a) and (b) use real water (or other liquids). Some children at this stage may not be able to pretend that a doll, for example, is wet when they place it in an empty toy bath.

TEACHING HINTS

1 Use the target words often during individual teaching.
2 Keep your sentences short.
3 Speak in statements rather than questions or demands. For example, 'Here's the wet one' rather than 'Where's the wet one?' or 'Show me the wet one'. You are showing the children something, not testing them.
4 If possible, let the children take the initiative, in starting the activity. Place the pictures (toys, etc.) near them and, if they pick them up, begin talking about them.
5 Store your individual teaching materials away from everyday classroom equipment. This will keep them special and interesting.
6 Give up gracefully if the children are having a bad day (or week!). If you persist, the children may be very difficult to interest on later occasions.
7 Keep your 'lessons' short. Stop before the children lose interest. Five minutes of individual teaching may be more than enough.

RECORD-KEEPING

Note the target words you have been teaching in a diary or day-sheet (p. 281).

MOVING ON

After a week or so try to find out how well the children are understanding the target words — use the activity on p. 187 to do this. Lengthen or shorten the period of one week, depending on the children's success.

Replace words which the children now understand with new ones from the list (or from your imagination). The 'First Words' scheme (Gillham 1979) will help to consolidate achievements at this level.

LESS DIFFICULT ACTIVITIES

It is difficult to tell when this activity is too advanced for children — you do not really know until you try to discover how well they have understood the target words. The activity on p. 187 will tell you this.

If they make little progress, return to some of the harder activities for developing recognition of sounds (e.g. p. 149–54).

Understanding words
Testing for understanding of nouns and pronouns

AIM

Children will show that they understand target words which have been taught to them.

SUITABILITY

The activity is suitable for children who
- appear to recognize some spoken words.
- have had target words demonstrated to them for a week or so (pp. 176–86).
- are at Stage 3 (p. 19) of our scheme for the development of communication.
   The activity is not suitable for children who have shown no sign of understanding words.

MATERIALS

Photographs and pictures of people, animals, and objects. The ESA Special Education Catalogue has a good selection.
Polaroid camera — for obtaining special photographs quickly.
Models of animals and objects. Toy furniture, with or without doll's house.
Dolls, Action Man, soft toys, and puppets.
A variety of boxes for hiding toys.
A box with a trapdoor (for sudden disappearances).
Some sturdy apparatus — chairs, benches, boxes — and cushioned matting for acting out the meaning of words.

PROCEDURE

Here are some activities which could be used to discover if a child understands 'dog'.
(a) *Acting on objects* Put two toys, including a dog, in front of the children. Ask 'Where's the dog?' If they point correctly approximately eight times out of ten, increase the number of objects to three. Switch about the positions of the toys so that the correct one is not always in the same place. Drop the two objects into a large cardboard box. Ask the children to 'Get the dog'.
   With the children watching, place a small cardboard box (or cloth) over each object and ask the children to 'Get the dog'.
(b) *Unpredictable opportunities* When tidying up, for example, hold out your

187

hand and say 'Give me the dog'. How much help do you have to give the children by pointing or looking in the correct direction?

(c) *Photographs and pictures* Photographs or pictures of individual objects can be used in the same way as toys or models in (a) above. Obtain a large picture with two or three different dogs in it (*Child Education* is a good source of these). Direct the children's attention to the picture by short sentences such as 'Let's find the dog' or 'Where's the dog?' *Occasionally* try pointing to a picture of something which is clearly not a dog (for example, a wastebin) and ask 'Is this a dog?' Watch for any puzzlement on the children's face, point out a dog, and then ask again. Is there any change in the children's expression?

(d) *Use of surprise* Basically similar to (a) and (c) above, except that this time the children make something interesting happen if they point correctly. The object can vanish through a trapdoor, for example, a bell may ring, or a light may flash.

TEACHING HINTS

1 Unwittingly, you may be looking at or pointing to an object which is the 'correct' answer. Use gesture and eye-pointing in the early stages if you think it will help, but make a note in your records if you are doing this.
2 Fade out any deliberate help (such as gesture) as the children progress.
3 Show them that you are pleased when they succeed.

RECORD-KEEPING

Keep a note of progress in a diary or day-sheet (p. 281) or use a word-record (p. 283) to note details of words which are understood.

MOVING ON

Move on to activities for encouraging the children to speak when you are sure that they understand some of the target words.

LESS DIFFICULT ACTIVITIES

If the children do not understand the target words you have chosen, return to the stage of demonstrating them (pp. 176–86). Alternatively, choose new target words which may have a better chance of being learned.

Understanding words
Testing for understanding of words which are not nouns or pronouns

AIM

The children will show that they understand target words which have been taught to them previously.

SUITABILITY

The activity is suitable for children who
- show some understanding of language.
- have had their attention brought to new words by similar means to those described on pp. 176–86.
- have reached at least Stage 3 (p. 19) of our scheme for the development of communication.
  The activity is not suitable for children who show no understanding of language.

MATERIALS

Photographs, pictures, and models of any relevant objects and people.
Sturdy apparatus and cushioned matting for acting out the meaning of words.

PROCEDURE

Procedures for testing the children's understanding of the names of things which can be represented by pictures, photographs, or toys are given on page 187.

It can be more difficult to test the children's understanding of target words which are not the *names* of objects, but here are some examples.

Understanding of action words

1 Stand the children on a gymnastics bench and say (the target word) 'Down'. Show them that you are pleased if they jump or step off.

Unfortunately this does not really tell you if the children understand the word. After all, there is not much else you can do when standing on a bench but jump off it.

Make the activity more of a test by working on two action words instead of one. Stand the children on the bench and say 'Down' or 'Sit' (assuming you have taught them both words).

If they carry out each command correctly about eight times out of ten, they have probably learned the words.

2 Sellotape a doll's house person to one of the cups of a pop-up toy. Seat a similar one on a trapdoor box. If the children reach for the correct toy when you say 'Dolly go *up*' or 'Dolly go *down*', let them carry out the activity.

Social vocabulary

1 Note if the children stop doing something if you say 'No' in a normal tone of voice.
2 Note if the children hand over something they are playing with when you say 'Please' (or 'Ta' or 'Thank you').
3 Note if the children wave or lift their hand when you say (but do not wave) 'Bye-bye'.

TEACHING HINTS

1 If you decide to use new apparatus for testing the children's understanding of words, give them a chance to play with it first of all. For example, they may not know that the pop-up toy produces an interesting happening.
2 Recognize when you are helping the children to pick the correct answer. Pointing with your hands or with the movement of your body is a way to do this. You can also point with your eyes by looking at the correct choice. The tone of your voice also discloses a lot of information.

It is natural and normal to give this help, but don't be deceived into thinking that the children are responding to the word alone.

Note any help you give in your diary or record-sheet.
3 Use as few words as possible when giving directions to the children — fewer than four if possible. Otherwise the children may not pick out the target word when you speak.

RECORD-KEEPING

Use a day-sheet or word-record (p. 283) marked 'comprehension'.

MOVING ON

When you are confident that the children have learned to recognize words that you have been teaching, move to activities that will encourage them to speak these words spontaneously. See pp. 191–211.

LESS DIFFICULT ACTIVITIES

If the children show no sign of understanding the target words make sure that you are not using instructions which are too long. Make sure also that you have given them sufficient opportunity to learn the words (pp. 176–86).

If they still don't seem to be learning, change to another target word.

Producing first words
The 'as if' technique

AIM

The children will be encouraged to use vocal sounds to communicate.

SUITABILITY

The activity is suitable for children who
- understand some words.
- make vocal sounds which sound like words but which cannot be understood.
- have reached Stage 3 or 4 (pp. 19–22) of our scheme for the development of communication.

   The activity is not suitable for children who are already speaking, especially if you want to improve the quality of their articulation.

MATERIALS

None.

PROCEDURE

Note any sounds which the children produce consistently. Do you think they are trying to say something with any of them?

   Could they be trying to say that they want something? Could they be passing a comment on what is happening? Note your ideas on a word-record (p. 283).

   When you hear any of these sounds in future, behave *as if* the children have said what you thought they said. For example,
- give them what they seem to be asking for.
- make a very short comment which carries on the sense of what you thought they said.

   If you can make no sense of the sounds, repeat what they have just said. Note what happens. Encourage them to carry on making sounds.

TEACHING HINTS

1 Keep notes of
    - *when*, or *after what*, each sound is made.
    - *where* it is said.

- *to whom* it is said.
- *how that person reacted*.
- what you think they were *trying to say*.

2 Do not worry too much about articulation if the children make very few sounds.

RECORD-KEEPING

Use a word-record (p. 283).

MOVING ON

When you can understand a few sounds that the children produce, move to
- other speech-production activities (e.g. p. 193).
- developing understanding of words (pp. 176–90).

LESS DIFFICULT ACTIVITIES

If the children do not produce word-like sounds, encourage them to produce a variety of vocal sounds of any sort (e.g. pp. 164–7).

Producing first words
The missing-words technique

AIM

The children will insert missing words in a sentence spoken by an adult.

SUITABILITY

The activity is suitable for children who
- understand a number of words.
- can speak, or seem ready to speak, a few words.
- are at Stage 4 or 5 (pp. 21–4) of our scheme for the development of communication.

 The activity is not suitable for children who do not understand speech.

MATERIALS

None.

PROCEDURE

There are several opportunities for carrying out this type of activity in normal classwork.

Poems and nursery rhymes

Pick poems which the children like and, if possible, ones with a strong rhythmic flow. Recite a line or two of the poem and then stop just as you come to a word which
- is on a strong rhythmic beat.
- or is at the end of a line.
- or is a word which the children have been heard to say previously.
- or is one of the words from the children's target list (pp. 176–86).

 Encourage any attempts they make to fill in the blank.

Stories

Action stories such as 'the great big enormous turnip' are ideal. So are others with a refrain. 'The little gingerbread man' is a good example.

 If the 'turnip' story is told to and acted out with a group of children, the word 'pull' will probably be supplied by some of the children spontaneously. Watch to see if the child you are concentrating on joins in.

 Encourage any attempt they make, especially if they produce words.

Singing

Songs are used in the same way as poems, but they have two extra advantages. First, some children seem to listen more carefully to sung words than to spoken ones. Second, a word missed out at the end of the line of a song will spoil a tune as well as a sequence of words.

Action songs should encourage even more participation.

The *Apusskidu* and *Okki-tokki-unga* songbooks (Harrop, Blakeley, and Gadsby 1975 and Harrop 1976) contain good examples.

TEACHING HINTS

In this informal kind of activity, try not to bring out target words by questioning or by telling the child to speak.

RECORD-KEEPING

Notes in a diary may be sufficient, but a word-record (p. 283) should also be kept.

MOVING ON

Move on to new target words when existing ones are eventually produced. When the children can produce about twenty words spontaneously, look at
- connected speech (pp. 225–36).
- developing comprehension (pp. 212–24).

LESS DIFFICULT ACTIVITIES

If the children do not insert missing words spontaneously, make sure that they recognize the word you want them to say (pp. 187–90).

If they do understand them but still will not speak them, consult the notes on children who do not produce words (p. 263) and on group activities (p. 204).

Producing first words
First commands

AIM

The children will produce words which act as commands, controlling the behaviour of other people.

SUITABILITY

The activity is suitable for children who
- understand 'target words' (pp. 176–86).
- use or imitate words occasionally.
- understand quite a few words that they hear.
- are at Stage 4 or 5 (pp. 21–4) of our scheme for the development of communication.

The activity is not suitable for children who show no sign of understanding spoken language.

MATERIALS

Benches, chairs, gymnastic mats.

PROCEDURE

Select target words which can be acted out by you and the children. The children should be able to understand them. 'Down' is used to illustrate the sequence of steps in this activity.
1 Go through a number of activities with the children acting out and saying 'Down'. Here are some examples:
  - jumping down from a bench or a thick activity-mattress.
  - standing beside a chair, then sitting down.
  - standing, then crouching down.
  - kneeling, then lying down.
    Lie/sit/jump down when you give the command 'Down', and make sure that the children do so too.
2 At this step, the children have to follow your command — do not show them what to do.
    Show them that you are pleased when they try to get it right.
3 Climb on to the bench, or kneel on the floor. Tell the children to say 'Down' (e.g. 'You say ''Down''.'). If they make any attempt at speaking, carry out

195

the action. They are learning to control people by their voice.

4 Later, pretend not to understand if you think their commands could be clearer. The fact that they are giving you orders may encourage them to make a better attempt.

TEACHING HINTS

1 It can be useful to have two adults working with the child at Step 3. One tells the child what to say, the other carries out the command.
2 Use short sentences — aim for a maximum of four words.

RECORD-KEEPING

Use a word-record (p. 283).

MOVING ON

When the child is successful at Step 4, introduce some other command words in the activity. Take turns to give orders. This could also be developed into a group activity using children who can talk quite well in addition to those who are just beginning.

Look at activities for developing
• comprehension (pp. 212–24).
• connected speech (pp. 225–37).

LESS DIFFICULT ACTIVITIES

If the children do not begin to give single-word commands, make sure that they understand the word you want them to say (pp. 187–90).

If they do understand them but still will not say them, read the notes on children who do not produce words (p. 263), and on group activities (p. 204).

Producing first words
Words for making things happen

AIM

The children will produce a word which makes an interesting event take place.

SUITABILITY

The activity is suitable for children who
- understand 'target words' (pp. 176–86).
- use or imitate words occasionally.
- understand quite a few words that they hear.
- are at Stage 4 or 5 (pp. 21, 24) of our scheme for the development of communication.

The activity is not suitable for children who show no sign of understanding spoken language.

MATERIALS

Down Box, Goodbye-Hello Box (p. 199), trapdoor boxes, jack-in-the box, pop-up boxes.

PROCEDURE

Select one or two target words which can be used with the above materials. You could use the names of objects which can be dropped into the first three boxes mentioned in 'Materials', or you could use action and social vocabulary such as 'down', 'gone', 'hello', and 'goodbye'.

Use the target words frequently when you and the children are playing with the various materials. Encourage any attempts they make at saying them.

Later, wait until they have said a target word before you let them activate a piece of equipment. For example, they might be allowed to let a toy car run down the ramps of the Down Box for a reasonable attempt at 'down'. They could spring the jack-in-the-box for a fair attempt at 'hello'. They could trigger the pop-up toy for producing 'go'.

Show them by your facial expression that you are expecting them to speak. If necessary, give brief directions such as, 'You say. . . .'.

TEACHING HINTS

1 Wait until the children have the idea of what is wanted, before you try to make their pronunciation clearer. You can eventually do this by pretending not to understand what they have said. Or you can make sure that they pay attention to the shape of your mouth as you say the word.
2 Do not give long instructions. Three or four words will be enough.

RECORD-KEEPING

Use a word-record (p. 283).

MOVING ON

When the children use a target word appropriately,
● continue to give them opportunities to use it — this will ensure that it is really learned.
● see if the word's range of meaning can be developed (p. 212).
● see if there are related words that can take its place as a target word (p. 215).
● look at the activities on connected speech (pp. 225–37).

LESS DIFFICULT ACTIVITIES

If the children do not produce words, make sure that they understand the word you want them to say (pp. 187–90).

Give them plenty of practice in making sounds for fun (p. 166).

Discover if they will use a hand-sign or point to a visual symbol instead of producing a word (pp. 238–42). If you resort to this technique, make sure that you continue to use the words you want them to say.

Illustration 2 Down Box (made from plywood)

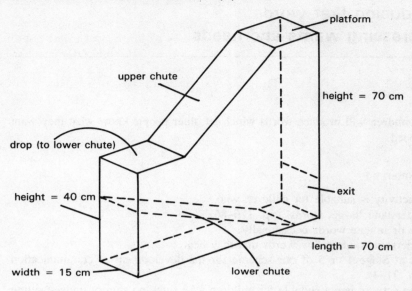

platform

upper chute

height = 70 cm

drop (to lower chute)

height = 40 cm

exit

length = 70 cm

width = 15 cm

lower chute

Illustration 3 Goodbye-Hello Box (made from plywood)

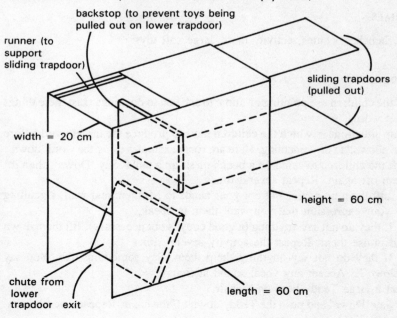

backstop (to prevent toys being
pulled out on lower trapdoor)

runner (to
support
sliding trapdoor)

sliding trapdoors
(pulled out)

width = 20 cm

height = 60 cm

chute from
lower
trapdoor exit

length = 60 cm

Producing first words
Expressing wants and needs

AIM

The children will produce words which let other people know what they want
and need.

SUITABILITY

The activity is suitable for children who
- understand 'target words' (pp. 176–86).
- use or imitate words occasionally.
- understand quite a few words that they hear.
- are at Stage 4 or 5 of our scheme for the development of communication
  (pp. 21–4).

The activity is not suitable for children who show no sign of understanding
spoken language.

MATERIALS

Chairs, benches, chutes, activity mats, large soft toys.

PROCEDURE

Note if the children use pointing or mime to ask you to do things. List these things
as target words.

Set up situations in which the children have to produce the target word before
they are allowed to do something. Here are some examples using the word 'down':
(a) Lift the children to stand on a bench or sit on a table. Say 'Down', then lift
    them off again. Repeat several times.

    Lift them up again. Put out your hands to lift them and wait, signalling
    by your expression that you want them to speak.

    If they do not say anything (a good copy is not necessary), lift them down
    and praise them. Repeat the activity several times.

    If they do not say anything, help them. Say something like 'You say
    "*Down*".' Accept any vocal sound at first.
(b) Seat a large Teddy bear on a chair.

    Say 'Down' and push the Teddy down off the chair. Repeat several times.
    Let the child join in pushing.

    Replace the Teddy on the chair. By mime or gesture, or by saying 'You say "*Down*"', encourage the children to speak.

If they produce any sound, allow them to push the Teddy down from the chair.

Do not let them push unless they make a vocal sound.

(c) Have the children sit at the top of a chute. Say 'Down', and let them slide. Repeat several times.

Seat them at the top again. Do not let them slide until they have said 'Down' or have made some other acceptable sound. Encourage them to do this by your expression or by saying 'You say "*Down*".'

TEACHING HINTS

1 Wait until the children have the idea of what is wanted, before you try to make their pronunciation clearer.

You can eventually do this by pretending not to understand what they have said. Or you can make sure that they pay attention to the shape your mouth makes as you say the word.

2 Do not give long instructions. Three or four words will be enough.

RECORD-KEEPING

Use a word-record (p. 283).

MOVING ON

When the children do use a target word appropriately
- continue to give them opportunities to use it — this will ensure that it is really learned.
- see if the word's range of meaning can be developed (p. 212).
- see if there are related words that can take its place as a target word (p. 215).
- look at the activities on connected speech (pp. 225–37).

LESS DIFFICULT ACTIVITIES

If the children do not produce the target words you want, make sure that they understand them. Look again at the preparatory activities (pp. 176–90).

Try to make the activity as natural or as much like a game as possible. Do not make it seem like a test.

Producing first words
Talking about toys

AIM

The children will speak target words that they have learned to understand.

SUITABILITY

The activity is suitable for children who
- understand 'target words' (pp. 176–86).
- use or imitate words occasionally.
- understand quite a few words that they hear.
- are at Stage 4 or 5 of our scheme for the development of communication (pp. 21–4).

The activity is not suitable for children who show no sign of understanding spoken language.

MATERIALS

Dolls, model vehicles, animals, buildings, people, and furniture.
Sand-tray.

PROCEDURE

This can be a group activity or an individual activity.

Catch the children's interest in the toys. If possible, let them take the lead in playing with them so that the activity is less formal. Then use the 'missing words' technique. Bring the child up to a point at which there is only one word which will complete a sentence correctly. Stop abruptly and encourage any attempt they make to supply the missing word. Here are two examples:

(a) A model town can be set up in a sand-tray. Opportunities arise for using vocabulary about buildings, vehicles, and position.

'Here come the cars. One for this house. One for *this* . . . '. [house]
'Here comes the lorry. Here comes the . . . . ' [bus]
'He's on the house. He'll fall . . . . ' [down]

(b) Dolls and soft toys can be used in games of make-believe.

'Take the brush. We'll brush Teddy's . . . . ' [teeth]
'Dolly wants some . . . . ' [juice]
'Teddy's going to jump. Ready, steady, ... ' [go]

TEACHING HINTS

1 Use short sentences — aim for a maximum of four words.
2 Use the target word while you are talking about the activity.
3 Make the activity as little like a test as possible. Face-to-face teaching across a table is not likely to be much good. Neither are formal, drab materials.
4 Avoid asking questions.

RECORD-KEEPING

Use a word-record (p. 283).

MOVING ON

When the children do use a target word appropriately
- continue to give them opportunities to use it — this will ensure that it is really learned.
- see if the word's range of meaning can be developed (p. 212).
- see if there are related words that can take its place as a target word (p. 215).
- look at activities on connected speech (pp. 225–37).

LESS DIFFICULT ACTIVITIES

If the children do not produce the target words, check that they understand them (pp. 187–90).
　　If they do understand them but still do not speak, the most likely reasons are that
- they see no point in producing them.
- the activity does not interest them.
- the activity is too much like a formal lesson and makes them clam up.
　Consider the following
- change the target words — there are plenty to choose from.
- make the activity more like a game — see Teaching Hint 3.
- say the word for them and ask them to repeat it, but do not labour the point.

Producing first words
Group activities

AIM

The children will speak in the informal setting of a group activity.

SUITABILITY

The activity is suitable for children who
- understand 'target words' (pp. 176–86).
- use or imitate words occasionally.
- understand quite a few words that they hear.
- are at Stage 4 or 5 of our scheme for the development of communication (pp. 21–4).

The activity is not suitable for children who show no sign of understanding spoken language.

MATERIALS

See 'Procedure'.

PROCEDURE

The class shop, baking, self-care lessons, and other activities all can be used for drawing out words by the 'missing words' technique. Here are some examples:

Class shop

Point to a bottle of milk. Say something like 'Give me some . . . ' and let your voice tail off so that the missing word is obviously missing.

Alternatively, pretend to have forgotten what you wanted to 'buy'. Say 'Give me some . . . ' and encourage the child to supply a word.

Self-care (dressing)

'Your socks are on. Here come your . . . . ' [shoes]

Baking

'The flour is in. Now pour the . . . . ' [water] You could increase the chances of the children's speaking if you let them hold the jug, but prevent them from pouring till they make an attempt to speak.

TEACHING HINTS

1 Use the target words frequently in conversation during the activity. This way they will be fresh in the children's minds when you encourage them to say the words.
2 Use short sentences. Aim for a maximum of four words.
3 Try not to ask 'What's this?' questions.
4 Try not to make the activity like a test.

RECORD-KEEPING

A day-sheet or word-record would be useful.

MOVING ON

When the children do use a target word appropriately
● continue to give them opportunities to use it — this will ensure that it is really learned.
● see if the word's range of meaning can be developed (p. 212).
● see if there are related words that can take its place as a target word (p. 215).
● look at the activities on connected speech (pp. 225–37).

LESS DIFFICULT ACTIVITIES

If the children do not produce the target words, check that they understand them (pp. 187–90).
    If they do understand them but still do not speak, the most likely reasons are that
● they see no point in producing them.
● the activity does not interest them.
● the activity is too much like a formal lesson and makes them clam up.
    Consider the following
● change the target words — there are plenty to choose from.
● make the activity more like a game — see Teaching Hint 3.
● say the word for them and ask them to repeat it, but do not labour the point.

Producing first words
Additional target words

AIM

The children will use words with sounds which attract them.

SUITABILITY

The activity is suitable for children who
- understand some words.
- may have used words occasionally.
- are at Stage 4 or 5 of our scheme for the development of communication (pp. 21–4).
   The activity is not suitable for children who
- have not been seen taking part in any make-believe play.
- do not explore objects.

MATERIALS

None.

PROCEDURE

Note if the children react strongly, probably with amusement, to a word that you have said. Note the circumstances in which this happens. Repeat the word and see if they will imitate you. Add this word to your target list (p. 178) and set up situations in which it is likely to be produced naturally (pp. 191–205).

TEACHING HINTS

1 Do not worry if the children's articulation of new words is unclear at first.
2 Continue to give the children opportunities to rehearse their new words to make sure that they become established.

RECORD-KEEPING

Day-sheets or word-record sheets (p. 283) will be better than a diary.

MOVING ON

Move on to new target words when existing ones are eventually produced. When the children can produce about twenty words of their own accord, look at
- connected speech (pp. 225–37).
- developing comprehension (pp. 212–24).

LESS DIFFICULT ACTIVITIES

If the children do not produce the words you want, make sure that they understand what they mean (pp. 187–90).

Producing first words
Talking about pictures

AIM

The children will speak target words that they have learned to understand.

SUITABILITY

The activity is suitable for children who
- understand 'target words' (pp. 176–86).
- use or imitate words occasionally.
- understand quite a few words that they hear.
- are at Stage 4 or 5 of our scheme for the development of communication (pp. 21–4).
    The activity is not suitable for children who show no sign of understanding spoken language.

MATERIALS

Pictures in which objects and events described by the target words appear. These would include: pictures of individual objects (actions or people); wall-posters in which a lot of activity is taking place (see Arnold, Galt, and ESA catalogues).

PROCEDURE

Draw the children's attention to the picture and talk to them about it. Encourage any moves they make to point out things, particularly if they try to speak.

Then use the 'missing words' technique. Bring the children up to a point at which there is only one word which will complete a sentence correctly. Stop abruptly, and encourage any attempt they make to supply the missing word.

TEACHING HINTS

1 Use short sentences — aim for a maximum of four words.
2 Use the target word while you are talking about the picture.
3 Make the activity as little like a test as possible. Face-to-face teaching across a table may not be much good, especially if your teaching materials are formal and uninteresting.
4 Avoid asking questions.

RECORD-KEEPING

Use a word-record (p. 283).

MOVING ON

When the children do use a target word appropriately
- continue to give them opportunities to use it — this will ensure that it is really learned.
- see if the word's range of meaning can be developed (p. 212).
- see if there are related words that can take its place as a target word (p. 215).
- look at the activities on connected speech (pp. 225-37).

LESS DIFFICULT ACTIVITIES

If the children do not produce the target words, check that they understand them (pp. 187-90).

Check also that the activity is not too formal, discouraging them from coming out of their shell. Scan the activities on pp. 191-205 for ideas on how to make teaching less formal.

Try different target words which may have a better chance of being produced.

Producing first words
Bogus information

AIM

The children will notice that they have been given wrong information. They will speak target words to correct this.

SUITABILITY

The activity is suitable for children who
- understand 'target words'' (pp. 176–86).
- use or imitate words occasionally.
- understand quite a few words that they hear.
- are at Stage 4 or 5 of our scheme for the development of communication (pp. 21–4).

The activity is not suitable for children who show no sign of understanding spoken language.

MATERIALS

Pictures and models.

PROCEDURE

Make a game out of supplying the children with information that is blatantly wrong.

Use it to introduce humour and to catch attention, as the following examples will show.

Looking at a picture of a farmyard

'See the dog?' (A cow is what you point at.)

Playing with soft toys

'Shoe for Teddy's *foot*' (Put it on Teddy's nose.)

Class shop

'Beans, please' (Point to a bottle of milk.)

Show that you are pleased if the children laugh or smile. You may be luckier. They may say 'No' or point to the correct object. They may even give the correct word.

210

Encourage any attempt they make to explain themselves.

TEACHING HINTS

1 Do not over-use this technique in case you cause confusion.
2 Use short sentences. Aim for a maximum of four words.
3 Make the activity as little like a test as possible.

RECORD-KEEPING

Occasional notes in a child's diary may be sufficient. Alternatively, keep a day-sheet (p. 281) for bogus cues alone.

MOVING ON

If the child can spot your bogus cues, look at
• developing comprehension (pp. 212–4).
• connected speech (pp. 225–37).

LESS DIFFICULT ACTIVITIES

The activities for helping children to produce target words (pp. 191–205) and to understand them (pp. 187–90) should be less difficult than this one.

More advanced understanding of language
Development of existing words

AIM

The children will develop a broader understanding of the words they know already.

SUITABILITY

The activity is suitable for children who
• can talk.
• understand a useful basic vocabulary.
• have reached Stage 5 in our scheme for the development of communication (p. 23).
   The activity is not suitable for children who can understand few words.

MATERIALS

See 'Procedure'.

PROCEDURE

Look at the children's word-record and select some words which can be understood in several ways. Table 7 gives examples.

Table 7 A basis for increased understanding

Word group	Example	Range of meanings and applications
Nouns and pronouns	Milk	Milk in a bottle Milk in a tumbler Coloured (flavoured) milk Hot milk Powdered milk in (and out of) a can Condensed milk in (and out of) a can
	Beans	A can of baked beans Hot baked beans on a plate A can of green beans Green beans growing outdoors and on Jack's beanstalk, in a picture
	Mine	Something that belongs to me and not to anyone else Something that I use, though I cannot strictly say that it is my possession ('my school')

Actions	Down	Put your cup down
		Jump down to the floor
		Lie down
		Sit down
	Jump	Jump down from a chair
		Jump up from the floor
		Jump across a space
		Jump over the top of something
	Come	Come here
		Here comes Mummy
		Will you come too?
Modifiers	Blue	Blue sky
		Blue eyes
		Blue train
		Navy blue
	Fast	Cars move fast
		Children run fast (but not as fast as cars)
		Dogs run fast (faster than children)
Social	Bye-bye	I'll see you when I come out of hiding
		I'll see you after dinner-time
		I'll see you tomorrow

Write the words you have selected in a chart like table 7. In the right-hand column write down various useful applications of the words that you think the child will not know.

Use the activities you have tried at the 'Understanding words' and 'Producing first words' stages (pp. 176–211) to help the child learn these meanings. Here are some examples using the word 'milk'.

Large pictures, full of activity Do the children know that a bottle of milk is called 'milk'? Do they know that milk in a tumbler is also called 'milk'?
Class shop Milk can be sold in bottles, in several types of cans, and in different sizes, colours, and shapes of cartons.
Trapdoor boxes (p. 190). Will a child point out a can of condensed milk so that it can be dropped?
Puppets Sooty (with a child's hand inside) is asked to pick up the milk. Will Sooty make the right choice when faced with the choice between a can of dried milk and a bottle of salad cream?

TEACHING HINTS

1 Make the activities as little like tests as possible.
2 Note the gaps in the children's understanding, and invent new teaching activities so that they can be filled.

213

RECORD-KEEPING

Notes kept in a diary should be sufficient, though a day-sheet (p. 281) could also be used.

MOVING ON

Continue to rehearse newly understood words so that they are properly learned.

Look out for other words which children may not understand as fully as might be useful to them.

Look also for
- new words to learn (pp. 215–20).
- activities to help growth of concepts (pp. 221–4).

LESS DIFFICULT ACTIVITIES

If children have difficulty with this activity, make sure that they really do understand the word in some context (pp. 187–90).

Try not to add too many new meanings too quickly.

More advanced understanding of language
Selecting new words to teach

AIM

The children will develop a broader understanding of the words they know already.

The children will acquire a more extensive vocabulary, based on the words they know already.

SUITABILITY

The activity is suitable for children who
- can talk.
- understand quite a lot of words, but in a restricted way (owing to lack of experience).
- have reached Stage 4 or 5 (pp. 21–4) of our scheme for the development of communication.

The activity is unsuitable for children who have only recently begun to understand words.

MATERIALS

See 'Procedure'.

PROCEDURE

Draw up a list of words which a child does say and sort them into groups like those in the table below.

Miss out the 'Words produced now' column if the child uses so many single words that it does not make sense to count them. Also, change the 'categories' that are listed if you can think of something better.

Table 8 A basis for vocabulary-building

Word type	Category	Words produced now	Possible target words
Nouns/ pronouns	Names	Me, Mummy, Daddy	Names of friends, teachers
	Body-parts	Eye, nose	Hair, teeth, ear
	Clothing	Shoe, sock	Coat, belt, tie
	Food	Juice, cake	Peas, beans, banana

	Household goods	Clock, bath	Soap, sink, chair
	House	Door, bedroom	Kitchen, bathroom, window
	Toys	Ball, book	Gun, dolly, bubbles
	Animals	Bird, dog	Worm, cat, fish
	Garden and country	Tree, swing	Flower, chute, mud
	Vehicles	Car, bus	Lorry, plane, bike
Actions	Giving and receiving	Want, gimme	Give, need, please
	Movement	Down, come	Run, walk, lie
	Spectacle/ surprise	Bang, gone	Splash, look, hey!
Sociable words	Giving and receiving	Ta, no	Yes, thank you, here y'are
	Recognition	Hello, bye-bye	What's that?, night-night, oh dear!
Modifiers	Place	Here	There, outside
	Position	In	On, under
	State	Hot	Wet, dirty

Teach these words to children in the same kinds of way that are described between pp. 176 and 211. Help them to understand first of all (pp. 176–90) then encourage them to speak.

TEACHING HINTS

See 'Teaching hints' in the exercises between pp. 176 and 211.

RECORD-KEEPING

Keep a word-record (p. 283) until a child can use about fifty different words.

MOVING ON

You will always be adding new words to children's vocabulary. However, by this stage, children will probably be using connected speech (if not, see pp. 225–37) and their growth of concepts (pp. 212–24) will be improving. Begin to look beyond the Early Communicative Skills ideas to the list on p. 243. This will give you sources of ideas for helping the children to develop further.

LESS DIFFICULT ACTIVITIES

This activity will probably be too difficult for children who have just begun to understand language. The first activities for introducing target words (pp. 176–86) will be more suitable.

More advanced understanding of language
Development of attention and memory

AIM

The children will retain increasing amounts of information on which they can be expected to act.

SUITABILITY

The activity is suitable for children who
• can follow simple verbal directions such as 'Close the door', 'Bring me the doll', etc.
• are at about Stage 5 of our scheme for the development of communication (p. 23).
  The activity is not suitable for children who do not understand spoken language.

MATERIALS

See 'Procedure'.

PROCEDURE

Make a note of the most complex instructions that the children can usually follow without you having to help them by pointing or by miming.

Using this as your starting-point, gradually increase the amount of information you give them. For example, you might ask them to fetch two things instead of one, or to carry out two actions in order.

Keep a note of progress and, when possible, increase the complexity further by asking the children to fetch a greater number of objects or to carry out a greater variety of actions.

If necessary, help children in the early stages by pointing or miming, but gradually fade this help out.

Here are some examples which make use of familiar classroom equipment and activities.

Class shop A child can act as shopkeeper and can be asked to bring two objects from the shelves rather than one. Later this can be increased to three or four.

Fetch and carry In an easy version of the activity the children can be asked to bring two objects which are close together, and not very far away from them on the floor or table. Later the activity can be made more difficult by increasing their distance from the children and from each other.

When this becomes too easy the children can be asked to pick up a specific object from a collection (as would be found in a toy-box or cupboard). Also, they could be sent to different rooms to fetch things which are there.

Dressing dolls Use either a cardboard doll with cut-out clothes or a plastic doll with 'real' ones. Tell the children to dress the doll with two specific items of clothing.

Do they choose the correct ones? If this is too easy, ask them to dress it with three (or more) specific items.

Waiter service Cut out pictures of various food dishes and mount them on card. Alternatively, make plaster models of various foods.

You are a customer in a restaurant, the child is the waiter or waitress. The imitation food is laid out on a table. Give the child an order for two items which the waiter or waitress must select from the table, and then bring back to you on a tray. Three or four things can be asked for later.

This game can be played by a group of children. In that case you may have to help some of the other customers to make their selections.

TEACHING HINTS

1 Do not hold back from pointing, gesturing, or miming when you give instructions to the child. After all, these actions are a normal feature of real communication. However, make a note that you are using them.

   Do not give this sort of help when you want to discover what words children can understand and how much information they can retain.
2 Remember that your eye-movements can fulfil the same purpose as pointing with your finger. Guard against incautious movements when you are testing to discover how much the child has understood.

RECORD-KEEPING

Keep notes in a diary or day-sheet (p. 281).

MOVING ON

Being able to pick up three or four items in the 'Waiter service' game is near the limit of communication covered by this manual. Check to see if there are
• any of the more advanced comprehension activities which are still worth practising (pp. 212–24).
• activities for developing production of speech (pp. 225–37).

See p. 243 for direction on development of communication at more advanced levels.

LESS DIFFICULT ACTIVITIES

If children are not able to carry out this activity, check that they understand the main words in your directions (pp. 187–90). They may have to be taught as target words (pp. 176–86).

More advanced understanding of language
Learning the names of attributes

AIM

The children will learn to understand words which describe objects and events.

SUITABILITY

The activity is suitable for children who
- can talk.
- understand a useful basic vocabulary.
- have reached Stage 5 of our scheme for the development of communication (p. 23).
  The activity is not suitable for children who can understand few words.

MATERIALS

See 'Procedure'.

PROCEDURE

Table 9 lists some of the words young children use to put objects, people, and events into categories.

Table 9 Early descriptive vocabulary

Category	Examples
Colour	Red, blue, green, yellow, white, black
Size	Big
Intensity	Hot, loud, noisy
Shape	Round, long
Quantity	More, a lot, one (or 'a . . . object/name')
Equality	Same
Value	Bad, good, nice, dirty

Draw up a similar table for each child you are working with.

Fill in the right-hand side of the table with the descriptive words the child uses.

Now add new descriptive words which would be useful for the child to learn.

Teach these new words in the same kinds of way that are described between pp. 176 and 211. Help children to understand first of all (pp. 176–90), then encourage them to speak (pp. 191–211).

TEACHING HINTS

1 Use the relevant 'Teaching hints' between pp. 176 and 211.
2 Do not try to teach too much too quickly. For example, do not teach several colour names at the same time. Establish one, then add another.
3 Be careful about teaching pairs of opposites at the same time. 'Big' and 'small' are obviously opposite to adults. However, this is not at all obvious to children who are just beginning to speak and understand language.

   Children will *probably* learn the more striking member of a pair of opposites first of all (i.e. they will probably understand 'big' and 'loud' before they learn 'small' and 'quiet'). This cannot be guaranteed, of course, but you can keep it in mind when planning work.
4 Look at the very formal method of teaching the children to understand attributes (p. 223) if they are not succeeding with other methods.

RECORD-KEEPING

Use a word-record (p. 283).

MOVING ON

You will always be adding new words to a child's vocabulary. However, by this stage, children will probably be using connected speech (if not, see pp. 225–37) and their growth of concepts (pp. 212–24) will be improving. Begin to look beyond the Early Communicative Skills ideas to the list on p. 243. This will give you sources of ideas for achieving further development.

LESS DIFFICULT ACTIVITIES

This activity will probably be too difficult for children who have just begun to understand language. The first activities for introducing target words (pp. 176–86) will be more suitable.

More advanced understanding of language
A systematic technique for teaching the names of adjectives

AIM

The children will learn to associate the sound of a word with an attribute such as colour, size, or shape.

SUITABILITY

The activity is suitable for children who
• understand twenty to fifty single words.
• understand connected speech but are slow to learn attribute-names.
• have reached Stage 4 or 5 of our scheme for the development of communication (pp. 21–4).
   The activity is not suitable for children who
• do not understand speech.
• understand only very few words, such as common nouns and simple actions.

MATERIALS

The choice of materials will depend on the words you want the child to learn. The example given uses Unifix cubes.

PROCEDURE

This is a highly structured approach which you may dislike because it differs so much from the more gamelike activities in the rest of the manual. However, there may be times when you feel that 'normal' methods are not working, and in those cases the method below should be worth trying.

   In the specific example which follows, a plan is provided for teaching a child the colour-name 'blue'. In the example, 'A' stands for 'Adult' and 'C' stands for 'Child'.
1 Place one blue Unifix on the table. A says 'Give me blue.' Praise children if they carry out the action, but help them if necessary. (You are assuming that C understands 'Give me'.) Move on after eight out of ten correct attempts.
2 Place one blue Unifix on the table. Just beyond C's reach is a pile of white Unifix. A says 'Give me blue'; praise for correct response. Move on after eight out of ten correct attempts.
3 Place one blue Unifix on the table; the white Unifix are now placed within C's reach. Question, praise, and move on as before.

4   As Step 3, only this time the white Unifix cubes are just a few centimetres apart from the single blue one.
5   As Step 4, but this time the blue Unifix is close beside the white ones.
6   As Step 5, but this time the blue Unifix is among the white ones.
7   Place one blue Unifix on its own in front of C. Just within C's reach is a pile of Unifix which are all blue, bar one which is white. A says 'Give me blue.'
    (a)   If C gives A the *white* Unifix from the pile more than twice out of the ten attempts go back to Step 1, then return to Step 7.
    (b)   If C gives A the single blue Unifix eight times out of ten, go on to Step 8.
    (c)   If C gives A a blue Unifix from the pile eight times out of ten, the exercise is complete. A is now ready to work out new exercises in which C will have the chance to demonstrate what is meant by blue.
8   As Step 7, only this time the single blue Unifix and the (blue plus one white) pile are only a few centimetres apart.
9   As Step 8, only this time the single blue and the (blue plus one white) pile are side by side.
10 As Step 9, only this time there is no single blue cube, just a pile of blue Unifix to which has been added a single white one.

TEACHING HINTS

1   Lengthen or shorten the above plan according to the needs of the child you are working with. There are no hard and fast rules of procedure.
2   Support this teaching with more informal techniques (see p. 221) which will support this formal procedure in bringing the attribute-names to the child's attention.

RECORD-KEEPING

Chart progress in a day-sheet (p. 281) or a frequency record (p. 286).

MOVING ON

If you have some success with this technique, try it with different kinds of attributes, for example, 'big' or 'round'.

LESS DIFFICULT ACTIVITIES

If a child has difficulty in this activity, try less formal activities for teaching comprehension of adjectives (p. 184) — the gamelike atmosphere may suit some children much more than a formal technique.

Work also at building up understanding of nouns and action-words (pp. 176–83) as they may be easier to understand than adjectives.

Producing more advanced language
Two-word directions

AIM

The children will produce two-word sentences to direct the activity of other people.

SUITABILITY

The activity is suitable for children who
- speak twenty or more single words, but have not been heard using connected speech.
- seem ready for work at Stage 5 (p. 23) of our scheme for the development of communication.

The activity is not suitable for children who do not speak.

MATERIALS

An activity mat may be useful.

PROCEDURE

Select a few action words which children have been taught or have been heard to use spontaneously. If possible, pick words which can be acted out, such as 'on', 'down', 'sit', 'up', 'jump', or 'run'.

Also select any words which you think they may be able to copy with very little effort.

Make up a game of imitation in which you say the words and then act them out. Encourage the children to join in the action, but do not worry if they do not produce the action word. Of course, praise any attempt they make to produce words of their own accord.

Next, have the children carry out the action in response to your command. Combine the children's name with an action word (e.g. 'Anne, down', 'Joe, jump') and if necessary help them to carry out the action.

Now decide what is to be the purpose of the two-word directions. Expressing words and expressing commands are two purposes which are not too difficult to draw out. Here are examples of each:

Expressing words Hold the child's hands and say, for example, 'Donnie, say, "Donnie, jump".' If you hear any attempt at (in this case) three syllables, respond by helping Donnie to jump up. As confidence grows, prevent children from

225

jumping (in this case) until their attempts at speech become more and more like the words you want them to say. Help them to make better efforts by exaggerating your own mouth movements and by making sure that they can see them.

If you have access to a speech therapist, check to discover if any specialized help would bring more rapid results.

Expressing commands Your aim is to make the child give a command to one of the other children or to an adult. For example, 'Donnie, jump' would mean that the child was telling Donnie to jump, and 'Anne, down' would mean that Anne had to fall down to the floor.

Encourage any reasonable attempt by making sure that the command is carried out. As before, be lenient with the early attempts, but try to make the children speak more clearly as their confidence increases.

Children seem to like this activity because of the power it gives them over people.

TEACHING HINTS

1 Do not try to introduce too many action words into a single activity too early. One may be quite enough until the children are in the habit of using connected speech.
2 If possible, use two adults in the activities. One helps a child give the directions and the other carries them out.
3 Use as few words as possible when you speak to the children. This will make your directions less confusing.
4 Let children use a shortened version of your own name when you are the person they are directing.

RECORD-KEEPING

Word-records or day-sheets would be suitable.

MOVING ON

When the children are able to produce connected speech during teaching, look for real-life opportunities in which the skill can be put to use. Look at pp. 229–37.

LESS DIFFICULT ACTIVITIES

If children do not produce two-word directions, build up their ability to give single-word directions (pp. 195–202).

Producing more advanced language
Words for making things happen

AIM

The children will use connected speech to give directions; these will make interesting events occur.

SUITABILITY

The activity is suitable for children who
- can speak about twenty single words.
- have occasionally produced connected speech.
- are ready for work at Stage 5 (p. 23) of our scheme for the development of communication.
   The activity is not suitable for children who
- do not understand speech.
- have only just begun to produce single words.

MATERIALS

Down Box (see p. 199).
Goodbye-Hello Box (see p. 199).
Small toys to drop into the boxes (e.g. cars, balls, bricks).

PROCEDURE

Down Box

Play with the children to let them see how objects can roll down into the box and then reappear at the exit.

Then introduce your 'target' two-word sentence. 'Car, down!' or 'Car, go!' would be suitable if you intended to jettison a car. Encourage any attempt the children make to give the directions of their own accord.

If they do not say anything, be more direct. Tell them 'You say, "Car, down!"' Encourage any good attempt by letting them push the car down into the box.

Do not worry too much about the quality of their speech until they are in the habit of producing two syllables. Later, you can prevent them from pushing until you hear clearer pronunciations.

Goodbye-Hello Box

The procedure is similar to that which you would use with the Down Box, though you would probably use a different set of action words.

Place a doll, for example, on the upper shutter. Say 'Bye-bye, dolly' and drop it into the box. Say 'Hello, dolly' and make it appear again. Encourage any attempts the children make to join in.

If children do not join in spontaneously, tell them to say the target sentence. Reward any attempt immediately by letting the doll drop.

TEACHING HINTS

1 This type of activity can be adapted easily for use with any other action toys. Clockwork cars, the pop-up toy, and a jack-in-the-box have possibilities for a range of action words.
2 If necessary, draw the children's attention to your mouth when you are speaking the target sentence for them. This may help them imitate the correct mouth-shape and produce clearer words.
3 When working with children with very poor concentration, leave the lower shutter of the Goodbye-Hello Box open. This way, the toy reappears almost immediately.

RECORD-KEEPING

A day-sheet or word-record (p. 283) will be suitable.

MOVING ON

This activity is near the top of the range covered by *Early Communicative Skills*. Look at the activities for developing flexibility of speech (pp. 229–37). If they are too easy, consult p. 243 for sources of ideas at more advanced levels.

LESS DIFFICULT ACTIVITIES

If the child does not produce connected speech, give more practice with single-word directions (p. 195).

Producing more advanced language
Group activities

AIM

The children will use connected speech to express needs and to give information.

SUITABILITY

The activities are suitable for children who
● can speak about twenty single words.
● occasionally use connected speech.
● are at Stage 5 (p. 23) of our scheme for the development of communication.
  The activity is not suitable for children who
● do not understand speech.
● have only just begun to speak single words.

MATERIALS

The choice depends on the activity.

PROCEDURE

Select action words which can usefully be connected to a variety of nouns. See pp. 179 and 215 for some examples.

Encourage the children to connect these action words to nouns (and other words) in everyday classroom activities. Here are some suggestions for developing connected speech during a baking lesson.

Baking

Use any opportunity to give the children examples of the kinds of sentence you want them to say. For example, you may well have to say 'Flour, please' or 'We need milk' in the course of the lesson.

Create circumstances which make it likely that the children will have to use speech. You could keep some of the ingredients out of sight. Or, you could ask directly, 'What do you need?'

Encourage any attempt children make to speak. Later on, do not hand over the item until you have heard two words. If the children do not do this of their own accord, try the following methods:
(a) Turn a single-word reply into a short phrase. For example, if a child says 'Milk', you could say 'You *want* milk?' This way children will hear you

229

using 'want' and 'milk' together. This may help them to use the two together in the future.

(b) Don't hand over what they want till you have heard an attempt at connected speech.

Keep this method for children who are definitely able to use connected speech.

(c) Ask them to repeat what you want them to say. For example, 'You say, "Want milk" (or 'Need milk, milk please').

At first encourage any attempt at connected speech, and hand over the thing they want. Later, do not hand it over until the words become clearer.

Be careful not to depend on imitation as a means of teaching! Follow a similar procedure with the following activities.

Shopping

Use visits to real shops (or to a make-believe shop in the class) in the same way as baking lessons to help produce connected speech. The different setting means that you will be able to use a different selection of words.

Unpacking the weekly shopping from a box at home is another useful activity. It lets children hear the names of a wide range of objects. These words can be combined with many action words (e.g. 'here', 'please', 'give', 'out') to let them hear simple connected speech also.

Meals

Use a real-life meal-time to encourage the use of 'please', 'thank you', 'more', 'enough', etc., connected to other words.

Make-believe meals can be used to draw out two-word sentences such as 'Teddy eat', or 'Dolly drink'.

Bed-time

Parents or residential-care staff can help draw out connected speech at the children's own bed-time. Action words such as 'wash', 'dry', 'clean', and 'off' can be combined with a wide range of nouns.

In day-schools, children can play at getting dolls and soft toys ready for bed.

TEACHING HINTS

1 Keep your verbal instructions quite short. This is especially important when you are saying something you want the children to copy.

2 Make sure the children like an activity and is familiar with it, before you use it to draw out connected speech. If possible, let the children take the lead in beginning the activity which you will use for developing speech.

3 Make a list of the names of any objects which children seem not to know in the course of the activities. Make sure they have plenty of opportunities to hear them if you want the children to learn them.

Some words may need to be taught quite formally (p. 223).
4 Don't make activities too babyish. Respect the age of older children.

RECORD-KEEPING

Occasional notes in a diary may be quite adequate. A day-sheet or word-record (p. 283) would be useful if you required more detailed records.

MOVING ON

These activities are at the top of the range covered by *Early Communicative Skills*. When the child is able to use simple connected speech, look at p. 243 for sources of ideas for more advanced work.

LESS DIFFICULT ACTIVITIES

If the children do not produce language during these activities, check that they recognize the words you want them to produce — advice on teaching these appears on pp. 176–90.

If necessary, help them to produce these words in more formal, individual work (p. 223).

Producing more advanced language
'Yes' and 'No'

AIM

The children will use 'yes' and 'no' appropriately.

SUITABILITY

The activity is suitable for children who
- can speak about twenty single words.
- occasionally use connected speech.
- have reached Stage 4 or 5 (pp. 21–4) of our scheme for the development of communication.
  The activity is not suitable for children who
- do not understand speech.
- have only just begun to produce single words.

MATERIALS

Pictures of individual objects.
Posters in which many actions are taking place.
Model people, animals, vehicles, furniture, etc.

PROCEDURE

Using the pictures or models as examples, make up simple questions which require the answers 'yes' or 'no'. For instance, 'Is this a boy?'

If children do not reply, give them the answer, emphasizing the 'yes' or 'no' — 'Yes, it's a boy', 'No, it's a tree'. Nod or shake your head to make the point more strongly.

If this does not help, try giving the answer in a quiet voice as soon as you have said the question, e.g. 'Is this a boy?'; 'Yes'. Encourage any attempt children make to say 'Yes'/'No' or to nod/shake their head.

If children succeed with this kind of help, fade it out gradually by whispering, then by nodding/shaking only. Finally, no help will be necessary.

TEACHING HINTS

1 Children may not reply because you are asking them a question that is too easy. Use the advice in 'Procedure' to let them see that you want them to *say*

'Yes' or 'No'. You are not simply testing their knowledge.

2 Many of the questions which have 'no' answers are bound to be silly. Make sure the children are in a relaxed happy mood before you ask these questions — if not, you may cause confusion.

3 Keep your questions short. Emphasize the important words.

RECORD-KEEPING

Use a day-sheet (p. 281) for noting progress.

MOVING ON

This activity is near the top of the range covered by *Early Communicative Skills*. Look at the other activities for developing flexibility of speech (pp. 229–37), when a child can answer 'yes' and 'no' appropriately.

Consult p. 243 for sources of ideas at more advanced levels.

LESS DIFFICULT ACTIVITIES

If the children do not use 'yes' or 'no' in this activity, try to draw out the words by asking them if they would like a drink, or their coat, or to go out, or something along similar lines.

Shaking or nodding the head would be acceptable — see p. 155–63 for activities dealing with imitation.

'Yes' and 'no' could also be brought into games of make-believe (pp. 168–75) into more general class activities (pp. 204, 229).

Producing more advanced language
Carrying messages

AIM

The children will carry a spoken message from one adult to another.

SUITABILITY

The activity is suitable for children who
- speak short sentences.
- have reached Stage 5 (p. 23) of our scheme for the development of communication.
  The activity is not suitable for children who do not speak.

MATERIALS

None.

PROCEDURE

Make up a message of three or four words and ask children to tell it to another adult.

At first the adult can be in the same room so that the message will be easier to remember. Later, messages can be carried to adults in other rooms.

For once, children who echo what you say to them may be at something of an advantage.

Example

ADULT: Go to Mrs Cook. Say 'Fifteen for dinner'.
CHILD: For dinner.
ADULT: Fifteen for dinner.
CHILD: Fifteen for dinner.
ADULT: (Sends child to canteen.)

TEACHING HINTS

Keep your instructions short. Emphasize the important words.

RECORD-KEEPING

Notes in a diary or day-sheet will be suitable.

MOVING ON

The children who can carry messages can probably tackle most activities in this manual.

Look at p. 243 for sources of ideas for work at more advanced levels.

LESS DIFFICULT ACTIVITIES

If children are unable to carry out this activity, make sure that they are able to produce connected speech (pp. 225–8) or even that they are able to produce single words (pp. 191–211). Make-believe activities (pp. 168–75) might also be suitable for preparing the children for communication with other people.

Producing more advanced language
Giving information

AIM

Children will use language to tell about things which have happened to them.

SUITABILITY

The activity is suitable for children who
- can speak about twenty single words.
- sometimes use connected speech.
- have reached Stage 4 or 5 (pp. 21–4) of our scheme for the development of communication.
  The activity is not suitable for children who
- do not understand speech.
- have only just begun to produce single words.

MATERIALS

Photographs of family, pets, and people at school. Other pictures and photographs which the child enjoys looking at.

PROCEDURE

Make up a few questions which require short answers of one or two words. For example, 'Who takes you to school?' or 'What would you like for dinner?'

Try to find a time for a short session of this activity each day. Keep it short unless children clearly try to prolong it: you want them to enjoy speaking.

If you have a collection of photographs of family, pets, or the people at school, there is a good chance that children will begin speaking of their own accord. Encourage this, and use it as a basis for more conversation.

Try the following technique if the child echoes your questions:

ADULT: Who takes you to school?
CHILD: School.
ADULT: Mummy takes you?
CHILD: (Shakes head.)*
ADULT: Daddy takes you?
CHILD: (Nods head.)
ADULT: (Normal voice) Who takes you to school? (Quiet voice) Daddy.

CHILD: Daddy.

*An echo of 'you' might well be given instead, but there's no harm in trying.

TEACHING HINTS

1 A Polaroid camera will help you collect fresh, personal pictures quickly.
2 Avoid questions leading to 'yes'/'no' answers unless you want to teach the child to use 'yes' and 'no' (see p. 232).
3 Try not to ask too many questions to which you know the answers.
4 Keep as silent as possible once the child has begun to talk. Adults usually say far too much.

RECORD-KEEPING

Use a day-sheet (p. 281) for formal notes or the children's diaries for casual ones.

MOVING ON

This activity is near the top of the range covered by the Early Communicative Skills Project. Look at other activities for developing flexibility of speech (pp. 229–35).

Consult p. 243 for sources of ideas at more advanced levels.

LESS DIFFICULT ACTIVITIES

If this activity is too difficult, look at the activities which deal with the production of first words (pp. 191–211) and early connected speech (pp. 225–8).

Language without speech
Hand-signs

AIM

Children will use sign-language to express themselves.

SUITABILITY

The activity is suitable for children who
- understand language (or mime, if they have severe hearing impairment).
- can imitate actions and gestures.
- seem too shy or withdrawn to produce spoken language.
- may be physically incapable of producing spoken language.
- appear to have advanced beyond Stage 3 (p. 19) of our scheme for the development of communication.

    The activity is not suitable for children who
- are making good progress in the use and understanding of speech.
- are physically incapable of fine movement of their hands.
- do not understand language.

MATERIALS

None.

PROCEDURE

Obtain information about the signs used in a variety of the systems in common use. For example, see Jones and Cregan (1986) and Somerset Education Authority (1978).

   Alternatively, make up signs of your own which seem to be more appropriate for the child with whom you are working.

   These signs are then used as 'target' words in activities such as those on pp. 191–211.

   The following technique was used successfully to teach the Paget-Gorman sign for 'orange' (see illustration 4) to a blind child who would not speak. It can be greatly simplified, of course, when children can see what you want them to imitate.

1 Adult opened out child's left hand and helped child to grip left thumb with right hand.

Illustration 4 Paget-Gorman sign for 'orange'

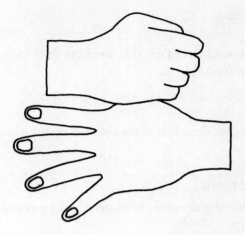

Adult held child's hands in position and said 'Orange'. A small piece of orange was fed to the child to emphasize the message.

2 As Step 1, but this time the adult did not hold the child's hands when they were in position.

3 Adult opened child's left hand and brought the right across to the left thumb, but did not help child to grip. Adult said 'Orange' (or 'Show me "orange"'), and praised the child for completing the action. A small piece of orange was given as encouragement.

4 As Step 3, but this time the right hand was brought only as far as the left forefinger.

5 As Step 4, but this time the right hand was not brought as far as the left one.

6 As Step 5, but this time the right hand was merely touched — no help towards the left hand was given.

7 As Step 6, but this time the right hand was not touched.

8 As Step 7, but this time the left hand was merely touched, not opened out.

9 No physical help at all, just the instruction 'Show me "orange"'.

TEACHING HINTS

1 Always use spoken language along with your hand-signs.

2 Make sure all adults who know the children (at home and school) are familiar with the hand-signs you are teaching.

3 Encourage any attempt the children make to replace hand-signs with speech.

4 Avoid making hand-signing an exercise in itself. Eventually the children should *use* their hand-signs, not just recognize them. They will let them express needs,

give directions, and give information. The child who was taught 'orange' in Paget-Gorman used the sign to ask for oranges and for orange squash.

RECORD-KEEPING

Note progress in a word-record (p. 283) when the child has begun to produce hand-signs spontaneously.

MOVING ON

Follow the 'Moving on' directions of the activities in which you are substituting signs for words.

LESS DIFFICULT ACTIVITIES

If children have difficulty in making hand-signs, make sure that they can imitate sufficiently well (pp. 155–63).

If they do not seem to understand that a hand-sign stands for a word, an action, or an object, make sure that they really understand spoken words (pp. 187–90).

Language without speech
Visible symbols (other than hand-signs)

AIM

The children will use visible symbols to express ideas.

SUITABILITY

The activity is suitable for children who
- understand language (or mime, if they have severe hearing impairment).
- can imitate actions or gestures.
- seem too shy or withdrawn to produce spoken language.
- may be physically incapable of producing spoken language.
- can recognize objects by sight (or touch, if they have impaired vision).
- are physically incapable of fine movement of their hands.
- appear to have advanced beyond Stage 3 (p. 19) of our scheme for the development of communication.

The activity is not suitable for children who do not understand language.

MATERIALS

The choice of materials depends on the symbol system being used.

PROCEDURE

Obtain information about communication using visible symbols. Blissymbolics and the use of plastic tokens are two examples. Information about techniques such as these may be found in Deich and Hodges (1977), Jones and Cregan (1986), and Somerset Education Authority (1978).

If necessary, make up your own system or an adaptation of one of the existing systems. In this way you may meet a child's needs more exactly. For example, raised Blissymbolics have been made by gumming string to cards, so that partially sighted children could recognize them more easily. Also, the chips in *Language without Words* can be made bigger than the original versions, and more like the objects they are meant to represent.

Use the signs as 'target' words in activities such as those on pp. 176–86.

The very formal technique for teaching the names of attributes (see p. 223) may be adapted for teaching the children to recognize symbols, if you have any difficulty. For example, it may be used to teach children to distinguish the target symbol from other symbols.

241

TEACHING HINTS

1 Adapt any technique which at first does not suit the needs of a particular child.
2 Make sure that all adults who know the individual children (at home and school) are familiar with the symbols they are using.
3 Encourage any attempt the children make to replace symbols with speech.
4 Eventually children should *use* their symbols, not just recognize them. Symbols will let them express needs, give directions, and give information. Avoid prolonged use of symbols as a simple recognition exercise that has no purpose in communication.

RECORD-KEEPING

Keep notes in a diary, day-sheet (p. 281), or word-record (p. 283).

MOVING ON

Follow the 'Moving on' directions of the activities in which you are substituting signs for words.

LESS DIFFICULT ACTIVITIES

If children do not seem to understand that a symbol stands for a word, an action, or an object, make sure that they really understand spoken words (pp. 187–90).

Beyond two-word sentences

Early communicative skills deals with the development of communication up to the stage at which children are producing their first simple sentences. If you are concerned with developing children's language at and beyond the two-word stage, the following sources should provide you with ideas for your own schemes of activities.

Bright Ideas: Language Development (Leibe and Quilliam 1984). A large collection of activities for mainstream pupils aged five to eleven. The activities can often be adapted for pupils with restricted development of language. Clear presentation of ideas.

Drama for Mentally Handicapped Children (McClintock 1984). The use of drama with groups of pupils who have learning difficulties. Takes account of a wide range of communicative abilities.

Language Development and the Disadvantaged Child (Downes 1978). Useful ideas for developing categories of spoken language such as nouns, qualifiers, and vocabulary of position.

Let Me Speak (Jeffree and McConkey 1976a). Sections 4 and 5 are concerned with developing the production of connected speech.

Listening to Children Talking, Talking and Learning and A Place for Talk (Tough 1976, 1977, and 1981). Advice on developing language for giving directions, reporting experiences, solving problems and so on. *A Place for Talk* is concerned with pupils who have learning difficulties.

Perceptual Training Activities Handbook (Van Witsen 1967). A large collection of activities which may be used for assisting cognitive and communicative development.

Teaching Language and Communication to the Mentally Handicapped (Leeming, Swann, Coupe, and Mittler 1979). The outcome of a Schools Council project. Covers the range of pupils in *Early communicative skills* and also pupils who have begun to speak in sentences.

Two Words Together (Gillham 1983). A structured approach to the production of early connected speech.

Ways and Means (Somerset Education Authority 1978), Volume 1 includes descriptions and evaluations of kits and other approaches which have been used with children who have begun to use connected speech.

Part 3

Problems in the development of communication

Problems

Children who do not appear to be conscious	247
Children who do not handle or play with objects	248
Children who lose interest in objects after they have been removed from view	249
Children who show few signs of purposeful behaviour	251
Children who do not understand that there are reasons that events occur	253
Children who do not understand the importance of the positioning of objects	255
Children who are unable to imitate sounds or the actions of other people	257
Children who do not take part in make-believe, imaginative play	259
Children who do not understand language	261
Children who do not produce single words	263
Children who use single words but not connected speech	265
Withdrawn children	267
Children who have difficulty in forming relationships with people	269
Children who are overactive	271
Children who are easily distracted	272
Children who behave impulsively	273
Children who keep repeating a word or action after it has served its purpose for them	274
Echolalia, or 'echoed speech'	275
Cocktail-party speech	277

Children who do not appear to be conscious

GENERAL INFORMATION ABOUT THE PROBLEM

'Consciousness' here is taken to mean awareness of one's own body and awareness that there is a world outside it. Without this very basic consciousness, communication cannot develop. Some of the most profoundly handicapped children appear to be asleep much of the time. Therefore the aim for people working with children who have this degree of handicap is to discover how aware of their surroundings the children are, and how much their awareness may be developed.

DEVELOPMENTAL STAGE

The development of the earliest levels of awareness is dealt with in Stage 1 (p. 15) of our scheme for the development of communication.

Children who are aware of their surroundings or who show any deliberate behaviour are at least at Stage 2 (p. 17).

GENERAL ADVICE ON TEACHING

Obtain a comprehensive medical and physical report on the child to discover if there are any activities which might prove harmful.

Make up a scheme of activities which will stimulate all the senses.

INFORMATION ON TEACHING ACTIVITIES

Teaching activities concerned with stimulation of the senses can be found on pp. 27-76.

The Educational and Social Needs of Children with Severe Handicap (Stevens 1976) provides a lot of useful information about teaching activities for the most severely handicapped children.

RELATED PROBLEMS OF COMMUNICATION

Children who have difficulty in forming relationships (p. 269).
Children who are not developing the early skills of thinking (pp. 248-58).

Children who do not handle or play with objects

GENERAL INFORMATION ON THE PROBLEM

If children do not handle objects and play with them, they may learn very little about the world.

Indeed, the ways in which children handle objects gives a good idea about their level of development even though they may be unable to speak. Young infants may do no more than take objects to their mouths. Later, they will begin exploring them with their eyes and hands. Later still, they will play with them in ways which they have learned by copying the actions of other people. Eventually, they are able to 'handle' (or 'make sense of') objects by giving them names.

DEVELOPMENTAL STAGE

The child's ability to handle objects develops throughout Stage 2 (p. 17) of our scheme for the development of communication.

GENERAL ADVICE ON TEACHING

Make sure children have an interesting range of equipment and activities which will encourage them to make use of existing skills and, thereby, develop new ones.

INFORMATION ON TEACHING ACTIVITIES

Teaching activities concerned with helping children to develop more complex methods of handling objects appear on pp. 87–108. *Let Me Play* (Jeffree, McConkey, and Hewson 1977a) gives useful general advice on the development of the skills of thinking which appear before the child is able to speak.

RELATED PROBLEMS OF COMMUNICATION

Relating to people (p. 269).
Other problems in the development of the early skills of thinking (pp. 249–58).

Children who lose interest in objects after they have been removed from view

GENERAL INFORMATION ABOUT THE PROBLEM

It takes time to learn that objects are not out of mind even when they are out of sight. If children do not learn this, they may not learn to recognize objects or search for them.

Children who are very young developmentally may not realize that an object continues to exist when they can no longer see it, feel it, hear it, taste it, or smell it. One of the first signs that they are learning that objects are 'permanent' is when they begin to follow moving objects with their gaze. With blind children, of course, evidence for learning would have to come from signs such as head movement, body movement, or arm movement.

Knowing that objects are 'permanent' is one aspect of the powers of thought which begins to develop before the child has begun to speak. As it develops, the child becomes increasingly able to recognize and search for objects.

DEVELOPMENTAL STAGE

Knowing that objects are permanent is one of the skills of thinking mentioned at Stage 2 of the section dealing with development (p. 17).

It begins to develop at a very early developmental age — as soon as children can look fixedly at an object held in the centre of their gaze. Later, their gaze will follow moving objects.

Blind children are unable to gaze at objects, of course. However, they may show signs of knowing that objects are 'permanent' by making searching movements with their hands or by moving towards objects which they want.

By the time that children are searching actively for objects which are hidden, it is likely that they will also have begun to understand some language and may even be producing a few words.

GENERAL ADVICE ON TEACHING

Work should be carried out in a varied and interesting educational setting so that the child is encouraged to explore his surroundings.

INFORMATION ON TEACHING ACTIVITIES

Teaching activities concerned with the development of object permanence appear on pages 77–86.

Let Me Play by Jeffree, McConkey, and Hewson (1977a) is also a useful source of ideas.

RELATED PROBLEMS OF COMMUNICATION

Children who have difficulty in forming relationships with people (p. 269).
Children who do not imitate (p. 257).
Other problems in the development of the early skills of thinking (pp. 248, 251–6).

Children who show few signs of purposeful behaviour

GENERAL INFORMATION ABOUT THE PROBLEM

Purposeful behaviour occurs when children discover that they can get what they want and make things happen by their own efforts.

Hand-watching is a very early form of purposeful behaviour which can be seen in young infants.

Later on children begin to explore around themselves, especially with their hands. In time, this leads them to reach out and pick up things deliberately.

Finally, children can be seen planning the moves which will let them carry out quite complex activities.

DEVELOPMENTAL STAGE

Children's purposeful behaviour begins with their earliest attempts to explore their own body and their surroundings. By the time they can speak the skill will be well developed.

It is one of the skills which appear at Stage 2 (p. 17) of our scheme for the development of communication.

GENERAL ADVICE ON TEACHING

Make sure that children have an interesting range of equipment and materials on which to work.

Play with them, using the materials so that they have the best chance of being interested by them.

INFORMATION ON TEACHING ACTIVITIES

Teaching activities concerned with helping the child to develop purposeful behaviour can be found on pp. 109–20.

Let Me Play (Jeffree, McConkey, and Hewson 1977a) is a good general source of activities for children who are not yet talking.

Purposeful behaviour will often be noticed among the other types of action which appear at Stage 2. Therefore some activities which are appropriate for encouraging early purposeful behaviour will be found among the less difficult examples of the sections of activities which begin on pp. 79, 87, 121, and 131.

RELATED PROBLEMS OF COMMUNICATION

Children who do not imitate (p. 257).
Children who have difficulty forming relationships (p. 269).

Children who do not understand that there are reasons that events occur

GENERAL INFORMATION ABOUT THE PROBLEM

Children have to learn that interesting sounds and movements do not happen by chance.

There are early signs that young children have started to realize this when they begin to follow moving objects with their eyes, or when they turn their head in the direction of a sound. Understanding develops as they reach for objects, and as they make agitated movements as if to make some interesting event (such as water gushing from a tap) happen again after it has stopped.

Later, they will touch an adult's hand when they realize that the adult has made an event happen, and later still they will hand over a clockwork toy, for example, to the adult so that it will be set in motion again.

Finally children will attempt to make the events happen by their own efforts. It does not matter if they are not successful — what is important is that they now know that events can be made to happen.

DEVELOPMENTAL STAGE

Children begin to realize that events have causes soon after they become aware of their surroundings. This skill has grown considerably by the time children have learned to understand and speak, and will allow them to solve simple problems about why things work.

It is one of the skills which appear at Stage 2 (p. 17) of our scheme for the development of communication.

GENERAL ADVICE ON TEACHING

Make sure that children have a range of interesting equipment and activities on which to work.

Play with them, using the materials so that they have the best chance to be interested by them.

INFORMATION ON TEACHING ACTIVITIES

Teaching activities aimed at developing the child's awareness of causality can be found on pp. 121–30.

Let Me Play (Jeffree, McConkey, and Hewson 1977a) is a good general source of activities for children who are not yet talking.

RELATED PROBLEMS OF COMMUNICATION

Other problems in the development of the early skills of thinking (pp. 248–52, 255–8).

Children who have difficulty in forming relationships (p. 269).

Children who do not understand the importance of the positioning of objects

GENERAL INFORMATION ABOUT THE PROBLEM

Children who have not learned that objects can occupy all sorts of positions in their surroundings will not be able to

- build a simple, mental 'map' of their surroundings.
- explore their surroundings.
- learn about how objects support, and can balance upon, each other.
- learn that objects can fall.

Long before they have learned the *words* 'near', 'far', 'up', 'down', 'under', 'through', and so on, children have

- been near things and far away from them.
- reached for things that are under other things.
- seen things passing through other things.

In short, they will eventually understand and use words concerned with the positioning of objects, because they have lived through *experiences* which make them real.

DEVELOPMENTAL STAGE

Children begin to learn about the importance of position as soon as they begin to explore their surroundings. This understanding will continue to develop even after they have learned to speak and understand language.

It is one of the skills which appear at Stage 2 (p. 17) of our scheme for the development of communication.

GENERAL ADVICE ON TEACHING

Make sure that children have an interesting range of materials and equipment on which to work.

Don't leave them unattended to 'teach' themselves. Play with them using the materials so that they have the best chance of becoming interested by them.

Give them every opportunity for physical activity which lets them find their way around their surroundings and for finding the objects in them. This can be especially important for blind children.

INFORMATION ON TEACHING ACTIVITIES

Teaching activities concerned with helping the child to become aware of the positioning of objects can be found on pp. 131–40.

Let Me Play (Jeffree, McConkey, and Hewson 1977a) is a good source of general ideas for work with children who are not yet talking.

RELATED PROBLEMS OF COMMUNICATION

Other problems in the development of the early skills of thinking (pp. 248–54).
Children who do not imitate (p. 257).
Children who have difficulty relating to people (p. 269).

Children who are unable to imitate the sounds or the actions of other people

GENERAL INFORMATION ABOUT THE PROBLEM

Children who do not imitate the sounds and actions of other people are not getting practice in using the behaviour which will let them communicate of their own accord.

DEVELOPMENTAL STAGE

Imitation of actions and sounds usually appears *before* children learn to speak, and *after* they begin to explore the world and play purposefully with objects.

The ability to imitate sounds and actions, and the ability to understand words often appear about the same time in a child's development. Imitation has very clearly developed by Stage 3 (p. 19) of our scheme for the development of communication.

GENERAL ADVICE ON TEACHING

Imitation of actions and sounds can be split into 'familiar' and 'unfamiliar' groups. 'Unfamiliar' actions and sounds are those which children have not been known to produce. 'Familiar' actions and sounds are those which they have produced already.

Imitation of actions can further be split into 'visible actions' and 'invisible actions'. Hand-clapping is a visible action — the children can see themselves carrying out the action they are copying. Patting the top of the head is an 'invisible' action as children cannot see themselves carry it out.

The distinctions between 'visible' and 'invisible', and between 'familiar' and 'unfamiliar' may help you when you are planning work for a child (pp. 155–63).

If you teach children to imitate words, do not assume that they understand them or will use them of their own accord.

You may not have to teach imitation at all. It can appear of its own accord as the child becomes interested in the world, explores it, and manipulates it.

Look out for signs that children have learned to overcome problems by themselves by imitating the behaviour of other people.

INFORMATION ON TEACHING ACTIVITIES

Teaching activities concerned with imitation of actions appear on pp. 155–63. Teaching activities with imitation of vocalizations appear on pp. 164–7.

RELATED PROBLEMS OF COMMUNICATION

Echolalia (p. 275).
Cocktail-party speech (p. 277).

Children who do not take part in make-believe, imaginative play

GENERAL INFORMATION ABOUT THE PROBLEM

Make-believe play enables children to understand the world better. It lets them explore ideas and feelings about objects and people without the objects and people actually being in front of them.

Children may play as if
- a toy were a real object (e.g. they make car noises when they are pushing a toy car along the floor).
- something were there which is not really there at all (e.g. 'drinking' from an empty cup).
- existing objects had a totally different form (e.g. a cardboard box becomes a bed, pointed fingers make a gun).
- they were someone else (e.g. mother or father, a policeman, etc.).

Make-believe play also shows that one object can take the place of another. This happens in language too: words take the place of objects and actions.

Failure to take part in make-believe play may be the result of unstimulating surroundings. It may also be the effect of severe learning difficulties — i.e. the child is *not ready* to pretend.

DEVELOPMENTAL STAGE

Imagination and make-believe are related to imitation. The children play with an object they have seen someone else playing with or using, and they carry out the same action. Therefore, look for make-believe play when the child is functioning at Stage 3 (p. 19) of our scheme for the development of communication.

The first sign of make-believe play may be the child pushing a toy car along the floor. Children are certainly taking part in make-believe if they hug or kiss some favourite soft toy. Round about this stage you would also expect children to understand quite a lot of words and also to be making their first attempts at speech.

Pretending that cardboard boxes are cars, or taking part in a lengthy sequence of play such as getting a doll ready for bed, will probably not occur until the child has begun to use connected speech.

GENERAL ADVICE ON TEACHING

If possible, take the children's lead in playing make-believe games. By all means stimulate their imagination by showing how objects and toys can be played with and used in different ways, but do not be so directive that they are discouraged from finding out the possibilities for themselves.

Do not expect make-believe play to occur before children can imitate the actions of other people.

INFORMATION ON TEACHING ACTIVITIES

Teaching activities concerned with make-believe appear on pp. 168–75. Other ideas for make-believe play can be found in *Let Me Play* (Jeffree, McConkey, and Hewson 1977a) and *Let's Make Toys* (McConkey and Jeffree 1981). Page 10 of the *PIP Developmental Charts* (Jeffree and McConkey 1976) lists some stages in the development of make-believe play.

RELATED PROBLEMS OF COMMUNICATION

Children who do not imitate (p. 257).
Children who do not produce single words (p. 263).
Children who do not produce connected speech (p. 265).

Children who do not understand language

GENERAL INFORMATION ABOUT THE PROBLEM

A child who does not understand language can make sense of the world only by handling and watching the things in it. When children can understand language, they are able to manipulate many more *ideas* and share the ideas of other people.

DEVELOPMENTAL STAGE

The most severely handicapped children (p. 15) do not understand language at all. However, as children develop their thinking at the top of the range covered by Stage 2 (p. 17) of our scheme for the development of communication, you will notice that they understand the occasional word. They may turn their head when their name is mentioned, or they may look out of the window if their mother says 'Daddy's coming home'.

At Stage 3 (p. 19) children clearly understand a lot of language. By this stage they will also be quite skilled at using the early skills of thinking (pp. 248–56) and will probably be imitating the actions and sounds of people round about them.

Communication continues to develop as children learn to speak single words and, later, to produce connected speech. At this stage comprehension is concerned with the learning of many new words and with developing deeper understanding of the words they understand already.

GENERAL ADVICE ON TEACHING

Use a 'target words' approach (pp. 176–90) if children are not picking up the meanings of words of their own accord. Use very short sentences or even single words when trying to draw children's attention to specific words. This way, they are more likely to notice the words you want them to understand.

Make it easy for children to connect the word you want them to learn with the action or object it stands for. It is easy to confuse a child who understands few words. Avoid asking too many questions. This makes teaching too formal and may discourage the child from becoming interested.

Comprehension is made easier in normal conversation by people's use of gesture, body-movement, tone of voice, and the direction of their gaze. Remember this lest you think that the child is understanding the words alone.

Later, the child has to learn that words have a wide range of meaning. For example, 'milk' is not just what is drunk from a cup. It is also something delivered in a bottle; it is produced by a cow; it can be dried granules; it will have a thick consistency if it comes from a can; and its flavour will vary depending on the can it has come from.

Comprehension is also affected by the grammar people use when they are talking. The order in which words appear in a sentence can make them more easy or more difficult to understand.

In general the best way to make words easy to understand is to use them in context and to use them for a purpose. If children see that they can get things done by producing words, this is powerful encouragement to keep using them and to produce more.

INFORMATION ON TEACHING ACTIVITIES

Teaching activities for developing the child's earliest comprehension of words appear on pp. 176-90.

More advanced activities appear on pp. 212-24.

The First Words Language Programme (Gillham 1979) is a sound practical guide which deals entirely with the 'target words' approach. *Let Me Speak* (Jeffree and McConkey 1976a) has general advice on a wide range of language activities. *Let's Make Toys* (McConkey and Jeffree 1981) has advice on techniques of teaching comprehension.

RELATED PROBLEMS OF COMMUNICATION

Children who do not imitate (p. 257).
No production of single-word speech (p. 263).
No production of connected speech (p. 265).

Children who do not produce single words

GENERAL INFORMATION ABOUT THE PROBLEM

Some children do not speak because they are physically incapable of speech. A speech therapist or doctor will be able to advise you about this.

Other children may actually be speaking, yet the fact is not recognized. Remember that a word can be

- a recognizable 'normal' word such as 'Mum', 'car', or 'juice'.
- a 'baby' word such as 'doggy', 'burny' (for 'hot').
- a distortion of a normal word, e.g. 'kal-eye-kaloo' for 'kangaroo'.
- a word that children appear to have invented, but which is nearly always used in the same circumstances.
- a hand-sign or other gesture (either self-invented or from one of the standard sign-languages).
- consistent pointing to a visual symbol (such as a Blissymbolic) especially if the child is unlikely to be able to utter speech.

Some children do not speak because they are very withdrawn (see p. 267), but others do not speak because people round about them do the talking for them (see the activities section pp. 191–211 for some ideas).

Finally, children will not talk if speech is beyond their developmental level.

DEVELOPMENTAL STAGE

Children's first words appear after they have begun to understand the language of the people around them.

The development of understanding and production of first words are covered by Stages 3 and 4 (pp. 17–20) of our scheme for the development of communication.

GENERAL ADVICE ON TEACHING

If you have been encouraging children to understand 'target' words (see pp. 176–90), try to draw them out in spoken language (see pp. 191–211). However, note that the first words children may speak are not necessarily those which they have been taught to understand.

Encourage any attempt children make to use words of their own accord. Look out especially for words which they like the sound of, as they may be more interested in using them.

Keep a note of words that the child has used. Details of record-sheets are given on pp. 281–8.

RELATED PROBLEMS OF COMMUNICATION

Echolalia (p. 275).
Cocktail-party speech (p. 277).
Problems in producing connected speech (p. 265).

INFORMATION ON TEACHING ACTIVITIES

Teaching activities concerned with the production of first words appear on pp.
191–211. See also *The First Words Language Programme* (Gillham 1979), *Let
Me Speak* (Jeffree and McConkey 1976a), *Starting Off* (Kiernan, Jordan, and
Saunders 1978) and *Let's Make Toys* (McConkey and Jeffree 1981).

Children who use single words but not connected speech

GENERAL INFORMATION ABOUT THE PROBLEM

A child who can produce between, say, twenty and fifty single words should be showing signs of wanting to combine two or more ideas in speech or sign language.

Connected speech enables children to carry out a much wider range of functions than is possible at the single-word stage. They can use connected speech to

- tell what they want.
- give directions and commands.
- tell what they have seen happening.
- carry messages from one person to another.
- give information.

As confidence in speech increases, they will also be able to use it to

- give yes/no answers.
- develop powers of reasoning.
- put themselves in other people's shoes and imagine how they feel about things.
- use their imagination in a variety of ways.

Some people find it helpful to make a difference between two-word *utterances* and first *sentences* proper.

An example of a two-word utterance would be 'my mum', as it would be difficult to say with certainty that the child was really making any difference between 'mum' and 'my mum'. Another example occurs when the child gives a list of object names (such as 'man, dog, boy') when looking at a picture — several objects may be named, but this is not a sentence as the child is not making any connection among them. Still more examples appear when children repeat a word, or when they join a real word to some apparently meaningless sound.

In first sentences proper, the connection of ideas is much clearer. In this case the most common examples are action words combined with the names of objects or people. 'Want juice' or 'Daddy jump' would be two examples.

The distinction between two-word 'utterances' and 'sentences' *may* be helpful when you are planning teaching activities for a child. However, the variation among children is so great that it is not sensible to make any specific recommendation.

DEVELOPMENTAL STAGE

Connected speech does not usually appear until the child has spoken single words. However, two (or more) word phrases may appear among the child's earliest words.

Connected speech appears at Stage 5 (p. 23) of our scheme for the development of communication.

GENERAL ADVICE ON TEACHING

Aim for children to put their spoken language to as many different purposes as possible. See the 'General information' section (on p. 265) for some ideas about what these purposes might be. This aim will be easier to meet if the school has varied, stimulating selections of activities available for the children.

When children have begun to talk, limit your own speech to the bare minimum necessary to keep them talking of their own accord.

RELATED PROBLEMS OF COMMUNICATION

Echolalia (p. 275).
Cocktail-party speech (p. 277).
No production of single-word speech (p. 263).

INFORMATION ON TEACHING ACTIVITIES

Teaching activities concerned with the production of connected speech appear on pp. 225–37. Look also at *Let Me Speak* (Jeffree and McConkey 1976a) and *Let Me Play* (Jeffree, McConkey, and Hewson 1977a, pp. 171–242).

For more detailed information on the functions of early language, see *Learning How to Mean* (Halliday 1975) and *Teaching Language and Communication to the Mentally Handicapped* (Leeming, Swann, Coupe, and Mittler 1979).

Withdrawn children

GENERAL INFORMATION ABOUT THE PROBLEM

Withdrawn children shut themselves away in their own private world. The most serious barrier to learning is their extreme difficulty in making contact with others, though many of them may also present additional problems. For example, some show compulsive, ritual behaviour such as ensuring that every brick in a tower is exactly in line with the ones beneath it. Other children fear change (e.g. change of room, clothes, food, activity). Still others will mutilate themselves by head-banging or eye-prodding.

DEVELOPMENTAL STAGE

Withdrawn behaviour is not confined to any specific developmental stage. People with severe learning difficulties may be withdrawn, but so also may highly intelligent ones.

It is often difficult to guess the stage at which withdrawn people are really functioning. To help you do this, look at the way they handle objects (see p. 248), or look for evidence of make-believe play (see p. 259), or discover through your teaching how much language they can understand (see pp. 187–90.).

GENERAL ADVICE ON TEACHING

Do not try to 'cure' the child's condition, but try to improve the level of functioning. First, make a note of any promising features in the child's behaviour which may help you make a start at teaching. The following ill-assorted list of 'promising features' is drawn from experience:
- a liking for oranges.
- an understanding of adult speech.
- the ability to read/'bark at print' (although spontaneous speech was hardly ever heard).
- being slightly less withdrawn in the presence of one particular person.
- being more willing to produce sign-language than words. (Remember that sign-language is communication too — don't hold back from using it.)
  The following advice may also be useful:

Get to know children well by observing them closely. Make a note of any people, events, or objects which seem to excite even the smallest amount of interest. Encourage children to come out of their shell more frequently. Do this by building on any efforts they make of their own accord.

Withdrawal and self-mutilation may also be severe reactions to boredom. Look very honestly at the activities which are being provided for children and question whether or not they are really likely to arouse interest. For example, has the same piece of equipment been presented to the child in the same way for many months? And would that piece of equipment be likely to interest a child who is not handicapped?

INFORMATION ON TEACHING ACTIVITIES

Use the 'General Advice' (on p. 267) when working through any activity which suits the child's level of communication.

Betty Van Witsen (1977) gives good advice on the educational treatment of a wide range of withdrawn children.

RELATED PROBLEMS OF COMMUNICATION

Echolalia (p. 275) and impulsive behaviour (p. 273) *sometimes* appear in withdrawn children.

Children who have difficulty in forming relationships with people

GENERAL INFORMATION ABOUT THE PROBLEM

Children's first social relationship is (usually) with their mother, who provides them with comfort and nourishment. Later, they learn that there are other people in their surroundings, and they learn to distinguish some of them — for example, they will hold out their hands to be lifted by people who are familiar to them. They will also play early co-operative games with them — for example, handing over objects that they have been holding in their hands.

Familiarity like this creates a good climate in which non-verbal communication and eventually verbal communication can take place. However, many children do not develop social relationships naturally and may be very severely withdrawn or very aggressive. This difficult behaviour can be a serious barrier to communication.

The child who does not form attachments and relationships will have difficulty in finding a place in the company of other people.

DEVELOPMENTAL STAGE

Social relationships continue to develop and change throughout life. Once children have become aware of the world — that is, at and beyond Stage 2 (p. 17) of our scheme for the development of communication — they will be taking an active part in forming these relationships. However, at Stage 1 (p. 15) they will make no obvious attempt at forming relationships actively and will be dependent on the adults near them for providing the earliest relationships of contact and comfort.

GENERAL ADVICE ON TEACHING

Children who are very young developmentally (that is, at Stage 1) will require contact and comfort in the forms of being held and talked to.

For more advanced children, it will be better to let them make the first moves in forming relationships as these cannot be forced on the children. Providing interesting activities and interesting equipment in a friendly atmosphere will encourage the child to become active and explore. This will give adults the opportunity to help the children develop their play, and create opportunities in which communication can take place.

The general rules of 'create interesting surroundings' and 'look out for the child's attempt to co-operate' also apply when working with withdrawn and aggressive children, though progress in forming relationships is likely to be very slow.

INFORMATION ON TEACHING ACTIVITIES

No specific advice on forming relationships is given in the teaching activities (pp. 27–243) as we are assuming that all communication is about forming relationships.

Teaching Children with Severe Behavior/Communication Disorders (Van Witsen 1977) gives useful information for work with children who are severely withdrawn or otherwise emotionally disturbed. Pages 57–112 of *Teaching the Handicapped Child* (Jeffree, McConkey, and Hewson 1977b) give useful advice on creating a climate in which good teaching relationships are likely to develop.

RELATED PROBLEMS OF COMMUNICATION

Withdrawn children (p. 267).

Children who are overactive

GENERAL INFORMATION ABOUT THE PROBLEM

Overactive children are always 'on the go'. They seem unable to keep their attention fixed on any activity for more than a second or two.

DEVELOPMENTAL STAGE

Overactivity is not confined to any one stage of development.

GENERAL ADVICE ON TEACHING

Individual work can be carried out in a quiet corner of the room or in a separate room where the child is less likely to be distracted.

Another way to channel the activity of overactive children is to set them tasks at which they are likely to succeed fairly rapidly. Keep them working steadily all through the task — do not let them daydream or wander — and show them how pleased you are when they succeed. Keep the lessons short, even as short as half a minute to begin with. Do not be in too much of a hurry to make them longer.

Overactive children may prefer lessons in which they have to do something with their hands, or in which they have to move about.

Check with parents and other members of school staff to discover if there are any circumstances at home or school which might be altered to make individual children less overactive.

INFORMATION ON TEACHING ACTIVITIES

Use the 'General Advice' when working through any activity which suits the child's level of communication.

RELATED PROBLEMS OF COMMUNICATION

Children who are easily distracted (p. 272).
Children who behave impulsively (p. 273).

Children who are easily distracted

GENERAL INFORMATION ABOUT THE PROBLEM

Children who are easily distracted have difficulty in keeping their attention focused on an activity. It is diverted by every passing movement, sound, or sensation, even when these would go unnoticed by normal children. The sight of someone passing by the window or the sound of a crayon falling on the floor are two examples of events which should normally pass unnoticed as part of the background, but which might easily draw the attention of a distractable child.

DEVELOPMENTAL STAGE

Distractibility is not confined to any particular stage in a person's development. It may appear in very young children, hindering them from paying sufficient attention to events going on round about them. It may also appear in older children, preventing them from paying attention to the tasks of normal class work.

GENERAL ADVICE ON TEACHING

You will often be able to catch a distractible child's attention by using brightly coloured, instructional materials, or materials which make a clear distinctive sound. These should be produced at the time of teaching only, so that the child's interest can be sustained over a period of time. However, you are also likely to hold children's attention if the teaching activity lasts for a very short time to begin with, and if the children experience success fairly often (even if you have to help them).

INFORMATION ON TEACHING ACTIVITIES

Use the 'General Advice' when working through any teaching activity which suits the child's level of communication.

RELATED PROBLEMS OF COMMUNICATION

Impulsive behaviour (p. 273).
Children who keep repeating a word or action (p. 274).
Overactivity (p. 271).

Children who behave impulsively

GENERAL INFORMATION ABOUT THE PROBLEM

Children who act impulsively seem to be driven into activity for activity's sake. Their behaviour seems to make little sense and is not directed at any purpose. For example, they may turn objects upside-down on a table, they may knock things over, or throw them, or they may haul objects down from your shelves.

DEVELOPMENTAL STAGE

Impulsivity is not confined to any particular stage of development. Any mobile child, irrespective of degree of learning difficulty, may act impulsively.

GENERAL ADVICE ON TEACHING

The following two approaches may be useful.

First, gather together a collection of material which the children are likely to play with purposely when they are not taking part in any individual or group activity. Posting-boxes, stacking-cups, sorting-trays, crayons, and modelling dough could all be useful. However, do not simply leave them around the room in the hope that children will begin playing with them of their own accord. Show the children how to play with them first of all. Bring the material to them to play with at the start of a period of free time.

Second, limit the children's opportunity for impulsive activity. Difficult-to-open cupboards and high shelves could be useful for storing teaching materials which are not in use, so that they are not available for them to respond to. Getting them used to the idea that free time should be spent in specific parts of the room may help to prevent them from upsetting work being done by other children.

INFORMATION ON TEACHING ACTIVITIES

Use the 'General Advice' when working through any activity which suits the child's level of communication.

RELATED PROBLEMS OF COMMUNICATION

Distractibility (p. 272).

Children who keep repeating a word or action after it has served its purpose for them

GENERAL INFORMATION ABOUT THE PROBLEM

This type of problem is called 'perseveration'.

Perseverative children have difficulty in shifting their attention to new activities, or in changing from behaviour which is no longer appropriate. They persist in repeating the same meaningless words, phrases, or actions like a gramophone needle stuck in a groove.

DEVELOPMENTAL STAGE

Perseveration is not confined to any specific developmental stage. Severely handicapped, non-verbal children may have the problem, but so may children of normal intelligence.

GENERAL ADVICE ON TEACHING

When children have to make a different kind of reply, or when they have to change to a new teaching activity, these changes can be emphasized by using quite different teaching materials. For example, you might decide that the materials for a new activity should differ in size, texture, colour, or sound from those which were used in the one which went before it.

You could also try moving the child to a different part of the room for the new activity, to break any associations of part of the room with one particular type of behaviour.

INFORMATION ON TEACHING ACTIVITIES

Use the 'General Advice' when working through any activity which suits the child's level of communication.

RELATED PROBLEMS OF COMMUNICATION

Impulsive behaviour (p. 273).

Echolalia; also called 'echoic speech' or 'echoed speech'

GENERAL INFORMATION ABOUT THE PROBLEM

In its most common form, echolalia is the echoing of speech which has just been directed at the child by another person. Frequently the echo consists of only the last few syllables of what the other person has said, though complete phrases (such as questions) may also be echoed.

People with echolalia seem to echo more when they are spoken to face to face than when other people do not look them straight in the eye or when their faces cannot be seen.

Other forms of echoed speech which you may come across are

- the echoing of instructions which have been given to children in days or weeks past — the children may sound as if they are giving a running commentary on what they are doing.
- the repetition of songs and poems — sometimes these can be produced by another person asking for them, but they may also be produced for no apparent reason.

Echolalia is imitation gone wrong, though presumably the child finds some reward or reassurance in it.

However, the echoing of poems or songs could be put to good use, for example, by letting the child perform *occasionally* in front of the children or members of staff. The ability to echo words may also help a child to carry verbal messages from one person to another.

DEVELOPMENTAL STAGE

Echolalia is a disorder of imitation, therefore it will not appear before Stage 3 (p. 19) of our scheme for the development of communication. In fact, it is most likely to be found in children who are capable of communication at Stage 5 (p. 23), even though their output of original speech casts some doubt on this.

GENERAL ADVICE ON TEACHING

Pay no attention to children's echoed speech; act only on speech which they produce of their own accord.

Echolalia may sometimes be the result of boredom and unstimulating surroundings at home or school. Check to see that children are being presented with activities which are really likely to arouse interest. Have they been working with the same piece of equipment in the same way for many months? Would that equipment be likely to interest a child who does not have severe learning difficulties?

INFORMATION ON TEACHING ACTIVITIES

Activities which have been used successfully with echolalic children can be found on pp. 193, 229–37. A very formal technique for decreasing echolalia is described in chapter 8 of *Operant Procedures in Remedial Speech and Language Training* (Sloane and MacAulay 1968).

RELATED PROBLEMS OF COMMUNICATION

Cocktail-party speech (p. 277).
No production of single-word speech (p. 263).
Problems in producing connected speech (p. 265).

Cocktail-party speech; also known as 'phatic speech'

GENERAL INFORMATION ABOUT THE PROBLEM

Cocktail-party speech is well-spoken connected speech which sounds very polite and very wise but is almost meaningless.

Children who use this type of speech are probably clever mimics who are copying the vocabulary and style of speech of adults they know. The politeness of their speech will gain attention and the approval of adults, even though it contains next to no information.

This emptiness of understanding is easily demonstrated by asking children questions about what they have been saying. They may latch on to one word in your question and proceed to build a new little speech round that, but you would not mistake this for a genuine conversation.

DEVELOPMENTAL STAGE

Because it is connected speech, cocktail-party speech would be covered by Stage 5 (p. 23) of our scheme for the development of communication.

GENERAL ADVICE ON TEACHING

Look at the functions of connected speech described on page 265. Note any of these in which the child is poor at communicating, and direct your teaching at including them.

Encourage the child to express ideas clearly, even if that means going back to one- or two-word answers.

INFORMATION ON TEACHING ACTIVITIES

Look at teaching activities concerned with increasing the understanding of language (pp. 176–90), and activities for developing the child's use of language (pp. 229–37). Page. 243 lists sources of more advanced activities.

RELATED PROBLEMS OF COMMUNICATION

Echolalia (p. 275).
Problems in producing connected speech (p. 265).

Part 4

Record-keeping

Day-sheet   281

Word-record   283

Frequency record   286

Type of record
Day-sheet

PURPOSE

The day-sheet is a general-purpose daily record of work. It can be used instead of the child's individual diary, or it can be used to supplement the diary.

One sheet (or collection of sheets) can be set aside for recording the child's progress through a single activity.

Alternatively, all activities which the child undertakes can be recorded one after the other on a single collection of sheets.

METHOD OF USE

Copy the day-sheet on page 282 or design one of your own.

Note the date and a short title for the activity in the first two columns. Use the third column to make remarks about the child's progress, or about any alterations to an activity which you decide to make.

File the day-sheets in the child's record-folder.

Illustration 5 Day-sheet

Child's Name ....

Date	Activity	Comments

Type of record
Word-record

PURPOSE

Word-records are used to note when a child produces a new word or phrase. They can also be used to record progress in learning hand-signs or other non-verbal sorts of communication.

METHOD OF USE

Copy either of the word-records on the two following pages. Or, design one which is better suited to your own needs.

Note the appearance of any words which the child has not said before. 'Target words' (pp. 176–86) and words which children have produced of their own accord should all be recorded.

Compare notes with the child's parents who should be encouraged to keep a word-record of their own.

Display word-records on the wall of the room if this will help during teaching.

File copies of the charts in the child's record-folder.

Stop recording new single words when there are approximately fifty in the word-record. Make a note of new phrases instead. Or stop this type of recording altogether when the child starts to speak in phrases.

Illustration 6 Word-record

Child's Name ....

Date when first heard	Word or phrase used	Date when first heard	Word or phrase used

Illustration 7 Word-record

Child's Name..

Date when first heard	Word or phrase used	Person (if any) to whom the word was spoken	What was happening at the time?	What do you think he/she was trying to say?	Dates when word or phrase was heard again

Type of record
Frequency-record

This chart is useful when you want to note how much progress children are making on a certain activity.

The activity for testing children's understanding of words is a good example. You may want to find if they can point correctly to a picture of a dog, say, eight times out of ten attempts. The 'frequency-record' lets you do this very easily.

METHOD OF USE

Copy the chart on p. 288 or design one of your own. Other examples of charts can be found in the books referred to below.

Note the activity you are using and the precise goal it is meant to lead to at the top of the chart.

Do not record the date in every available box in the main body of the chart. One entry per lesson will be enough.

The 'score' boxes appear in groups of five. This makes it easier to keep track of how many times the activity has been carried out in any one lesson.

Score with a '+' or a '1' when the children succeed with an attempt, and with a '0' when they do not.

Sometimes the children's attempts cannot be scored clearly as '+' or '0'. For example, they might deserve an in-between mark for an attempt at imitating a sound or action.

In these cases you could give them marks out of 2 or 4, for instance, instead of a '+' or '0'. Here are two examples:

Marks out of 2

Score	Meaning
0	Wrong
1	Nearly correct
2	Correct

Marks out of 4

Score	Meaning
0	No attempt
1	Wrong attempt
2	Poor attempt
3	Good attempt
4	Correct

Add any comments about the children, or about the activity, in the spaces below the score boxes.

File the charts in the child's record-folder.

For further reference on charting pupils using frequency-records and similar charts, see Jeffree, McConkey, and Hewson (1977b), Watson (1973), and Neisworth and Smith (1973).

Illustration 8 Frequency-record

Child's Name ....

Teaching Activity ....

Goal of the Activity ....

....

Date(s)					
Score					

Comments:

Date(s)					
Score					

Comments:

Date(s)					
Score					

Comments:

Date(s)					
Score					

Comments:

Date(s)					
Score					

Comments:

288

References

Anderson, C. (1983) *Feeding: A Guide to Assessment and Intervention with Handicapped Children*, Glasgow: Jordanhill College Sales and Publications.

Barrett, M.D. (1980) 'Early Pragmatic Development', paper presented at the Conference of the Developmental Psychology Section, British Psychological Society, Edinburgh.

Bryen, D.N. and Joyce, D.G. (1985) 'Language intervention with the severely handicapped: a decade of research', *Journal of Special Education*, 19(1): 7–39.

Dale, P.S. (1980) 'Is early pragmatic development measurable?' *Journal of Child Language*, 7(1): 1–12.

Deich, R.F. and Hodges, P.M. (1977) *Language Without Words*, London: Souvenir Press.

Dore, J. (1975) 'Holophrases, speech acts and language universals', *Journal of Child Language*, 2(1): 21–40.

Downes, G. (1978) *Language Development and the Disadvantaged Child*, Edinburgh: Holmes McDougall.

Education (Handicapped Children) Act 1970.

Education (Mentally Handicapped Children) (Scotland) Act 1974.

Finnie, N.R. (1974) *Handling the Young Cerebral Palsied Child at Home*, London: Heinemann.

Gillham, B. (1979) *The First Words Language Programme*, London: Allen and Unwin.

Gillham, B. (1983) *Two Words Together*, London: Allen and Unwin.

Gunzburg, H.C. (1966) *Progress Assessment Charts*, London: MENCAP.

Halliday, M.A.K. (1975) *Learning How to Mean*, London: Edward Arnold.

Harrop, B. (1976) *Okki-tokki-unga*, London: A. & C. Black.

Harrop, B., Blakeley, P., and Gadsby, D. (1975) *Apusskidu*, London: A. & C. Black.

Horn, R.E., Nicol, E.H., Kleinmann, J.C., and Grace, M.G. (1969) *Information Mapping for Learning and Reference*, Cambridge, Mass.: Information Resources.

Jeffree, D.M. and McConkey, R. (1976a) *Let Me Speak*, London: Souvenir Press.

Jeffree, D.M. and McConkey, R. (1976b) *PIP Developmental Charts*, London: Hodder and Stoughton.

Jeffree, D.M., McConkey, R., and Hewson, S. (1977a) *Let Me Play*, London: Souvenir Press.

Jeffree, D.M., McConkey, R., and Hewson, S. (1977a) *Let Me Play*, London: Souvenir Press.

Jeffree, D.M., McConkey, R., and Hewson, S. (1977b) *Teaching the Handicapped Child*, London: Souvenir Press.

Jones, P.R. and Cregan, A. (1986) *Sign and Symbol Communication for Mentally Handicapped People*, London: Croom Helm.

Kiernan, C., Jordan, R., and Saunders, C. (1978) *Starting Off*, London: Souvenir Press.

Leeming, K., Swann, W., Coupe, J., and Mittler, P. (1979) *Teaching Language and Communication to the Mentally Handicapped*, London: Evans/Methuen Educational.

Leibe, F. and Quilliam, S. (1984) *Bright Ideas: Language Development*, Leamington Spa: Scholastic Publications.

McClintock, A.B. (1984) *Drama for Mentally Handicapped Children*, London: Souvenir Press.

McConkey, R. (1984) *Learning to Pretend*, Dublin: St Michael's House Research (videotape).

McConkey, R. and Jeffree, D.M. (1981) *Let's Make Toys*, London: Souvenir Press.

McConkey, R. and Price, P. (1986) *Let's Talk*, London: Souvenir Press.

Nakazima, S. (1975) 'Phonemicization and symbolization in language development', in Lenneberg, E.H. and Lenneberg, E. (eds) *Foundations of Language Development*, vol. 1, New York: Academic Press: 181–7.

Neisworth, J.T. and Smith, R.M. (1973) *Modifying Retarded Behavior*, Boston: Houghton Mifflin.

Piaget, J. (1936) *The Origins of Intelligence in Children* (1952 translation), New York: International Universities Press.

Piaget, J. (1937) *The Construction of Reality in the Child* (1954 translation), New York: Basic Books.

Piaget, J. (1969) *The Science of Education and the Psychology of the Child*, New York: Viking.

Sloane, H.N. and Macaulay, B.D. (eds) (1968) *Operant Procedures in Remedial Speech and Language Training*, Boston: Houghton Mifflin.

Snyder, L. (1975) 'Pragmatics in language disabled children', unpublished PhD dissertation: Department of Speech Pathology and Audiology, University of Colorado.

Somerset Education Authority (1978) *Ways and Means*, Houndmills: Globe Education.

Stevens, M. (1976) *The Educational and Social Needs of Children with Severe Handicap*, London: Edward Arnold.

Tager-Flusberg, H. (1985) 'Putting words together: morphology and syntax in the preschool years', in Gleason, J.R. (ed.) *The Development of Language*, Columbus: Merrill: 139–71.

Tough, J. (1976) *Listening to Children Talking*, Cardiff: Drake.

Tough, J. (1977) *Talking and Learning*, Cardiff: Drake.

Tough, J. (1981) *A Place for Talk*, London: Ward Lock Educational.

Trevarthen, C. (1977) 'Descriptive analysis of infant communicative behaviour', in Schaffer, H.R. (ed.) *Studies in Mother-Infant Interaction*, London: Academic Press: 227–70.

Uzgiris, I.C. and Hunt, J. McV. (1975) *Assessment in Infancy*, Champaign:

University of Illinois Press.

Van Witsen, B. (1967) *Perceptual Training Activities Handbook*, New York: Teachers College Press.

Van Witsen, B. (1977) *Teaching Children with Severe Behavior/Communication Disorders*, New York: Teachers College Press.

Warner, J. (1981) *Helping the Handicapped Child with Early Feeding*, Winslow, Bucks.: PTM.

Watson, L.S. Jnr (1973) *Child Behavior Modification*, Oxford: Pergamon.

Index

Assessment 11

Behaving purposefully 18, 109-20, 251
Beyond two-word sentences 243

Cause-effect behaviour 18, 121-30, 253
Cocktail-party speech 277
Communication, activities 25-242;
    development 13-24; language without
    speech 238-42; problems 245-77
Comprehension of words, advanced 23,
    212-24, 261; basic 19, 176-90, 261
Connected speech 23, 225-38, 243, 265

Distractible children 272

Echolalia, 'echoed speech' 275

First words 21, 191-211, 263-66

Handling objects 18, 77-86, 248

Imaginative play 168-75, 259
Imitation, general information 19, 257;
    actions and gestures 19, 155-63;
    vocal sounds 19, 164-7
Impulsive children 273

Make-believe 168-75, 259
Making things happen 18, 121-30, 253
Means-end behaviour 18, 109-20, 251

Object-permanence 18, 77-86, 249

Object relations 18, 131-40, 255
Overactive children 271

Perseveration 274
Phatic speech 277
Position, understanding of 18. 131-40,
    255
Producing speech 21, 191-211, 263-6
Profound learning difficulties 15, 247

Record-forms 279-87
Repetition of words 274-6

Sign language 238-40
Sounds, production of 20, 164-7;
    recognition and understanding 18,
    141-55
Speech, connected 23, 225-38; 265;
    production 21, 191-211, 263-6
Stimulation, hearing 16, 27-40;
    movement 16, 57-66; smell 16,
    67-74; taste 16, 75-6; touch 16,
    49-56; vision 16, 41-8

Two-word sentences 23, 225-38, 243,
    265

Understanding words 19, 176-90, 261

Watching and finding things 18, 77-86,
    249
Withdrawn children 267